the REGENERATIVE MEDICINE in ORTHOPAEDICS

Browse Timeo books catalogue
on www.griffineditore.it or scan the QR Code

THE REGENERATIVE MEDICINE IN ORTHOPAEDICS

Scientific coordinator: Professor Sandro Giannini
Editing and proofreading: Maria Camillo
Design and layout Marco Redaelli

Printing: Starprint srl
1st edition – English version March 2022

PUBLISHER
Griffin srl unipersonale
Via cavalluccio 2B - 22060 - Carimate (Como)
Tel. 031.789085
customerservice@griffineditore.it
www.griffineditore.it

ISBN 978-88-97162-94-0

PREFACE

Biological repair of the musculoskeletal system is one of the main purposes in orthopedics and traumatology.
In recent years, these two disciplines have had a particular development with the creation and use of new materials, new designs of synthetic media, prosthetic implants, and new instruments for their applications.
The research to reconstruct the damaged tissues has always been the mirage of the orthopedic surgeon for which regenerative medicine has progressively developed, intending to get to repair bones, cartilage, tendons, muscles, and skin.
With the publication of this book, we wanted to collect the developed experience of years at the Rizzoli Institute with the integration between research laboratories and clinical divisions and with the experience of other laboratories and surgeons of national and international importance.
After an introductory part of basic science related to the biological materials used: stem cells, platelet aggregates and scaffolds, some cell isolation systems are presented. Subsequently, animal studies and the most common clinical applications are presented, including bone repair, cartilage, muscle, and tendons. In addition to the various surgical treatments, the effect of biophysical stimulation on tissue regeneration is also treated.
I want to thank all the colleagues who have agreed to participate in the realization of this volume by writing articles that collect an experience of years of work.
I hope that this book that has the advantage of collecting essential science works, systems of implant products, and the various clinical applications may be of interest to those who approach regenerative medicine and to the most experienced.
In particular, I want to thank the DIBIDEM department of the Alma Mater University of Bologna, the Italian Society of Orthopedics and Traumatology (SIOT), the Rizzoli Orthopedic Institute of Bologna, and the Carlo Rizzoli Foundation for motor sciences, who sponsored the event that led to the creation of the book.

Sandro Giannini
Professor Emeritus
University of Bologna

SCIENTIFIC COORDINATOR

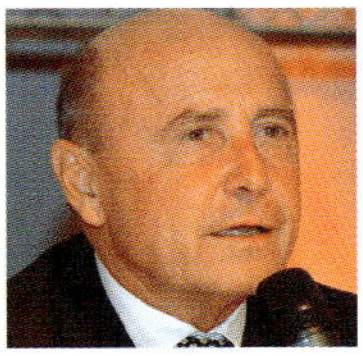

Professor Sandro Giannini

Full Professor in Orthopaedics and Traumatology, University of Bologna, Italy

Director of 1st Clinic of Orthopaedics and Traumatology, Rizzoli Orthopaedic Institute, Bologna, Italy.

Director of the Laboratory of Gait Analysis, Rizzoli Orthopaedic Institute, Bologna, Italy.

Director of the Department of Anatomical Sciences and Musculoskeletal Apparatus, Bologna, Italy

Director of the Residency program in Orthopaedics and Traumatology, University of Bologna, Italy

Director of the Residency program in Physical Medicine and Rehabilitation, University of Bologna, Italy

Director of the Graduation program in Podiatry, University of Bologna, Italy

Director of the Master degree course in Orthopaedics and Trauma Nursing, University of Bologna, Italy

Director of the Course in Microsurgery, University of Bologna, Italy

President of Orthopaedics and Traumatology Full Professors Collegium

Board Member of the International Society of Orthopaedic Center (ISOC)

Directory Board of the European Foot and Ankle Society (EFAS).

President of the International Federation of Foot and Ankle Societies (IFFAS)

Now Professor Emeritus, University of Bologna, Italy

Member of the European Foot and Ankle Society (EFAS), Member of the American Academy of Orthopaedic Surgeons (AAOS), Onorary Member of the American College of Foot and Ankle Surgeons (ACFAS), Member of European Federation of Orthopaedic Research Societies (EFORT), International Cartilage Repair Society (ICRS), Onorary member of the American College of Foot and Ankle Surgeons and of Brazilian Society of Medicine and Surgery of the Foot, member of Italian Foot and Ankle Society (SICP).

His career has been dedicated to constant research in the field of orthopaedics and traumatology, publishing more than 400 scientific papers (total h-index 54, source: Scopus). During his long practice he went deep into the innovation of many different fields of orthopaedic surgery, creating a bioabsorbable devices for the surgical treatment of the flat foot, the "one step technique" for cartilage repair, and a new design ankle prosthesis. In addition he is considered a pioneer in the field of bipolar fresh osteochondral allografts.

Sandro Giannini received several prizes and honours: the institution of the Sandro Giannini Prize, awarded at the International Federation of Foot and Ankle Societies (IFFAS) Meeting, the Memorial K. Johnson Award received from American Academy of Orthopaedic Surgeons, USA, the Guildal Award from the Danish Orthopaedic Society.

INDEX

CHAPTER 1

BONE MARROW BLOOD: TREATMENT OF FOCAL OSTEOCHONDRAL LESIONS

Andrea Pantalone, Danilo Bruni, Federico Del Gusto, Pietro Rao, Roberto Buda

Orthopaedic and Traumatological Clinic, Ss Annunziata Chieti Hospital

Department of Medicine and Aging Sciences, University "G. d'Annunzio" Chieti-Pescara

Introduction

Osteochondral lesions (OC) are defects of the cartilage surface and underlying subchondral bone; the most affected joints are the knee and ankle [1,2]. In the knee, they are concentrated at the level of the femoral condyles and the patellofemoral joint; in the ankle, the majority of these lesions occur at the level of the talar dome, while a localization at a tibiofibular mortise level is rarely observed [3]. The osteochondral lesions of the tibiofibular mortise are much rarer and less frequent than those of the talar dome, with a ratio ranging from 1:14 to 1:20. This is believed to be due to the anatomical conformation of the tibiofibular mortise itself, as its concave articular surface, as opposed to the convex one of the talar dome, is more effective in absorbing redistributing the different mechanical stresses on a surface of greater amplitude. In addition, compared to the talar dome, the hyaline articular cartilage in the tibial plateau is thicker. These two biomechanical characteristics give it greater strength and a lower susceptibility to osteochondral lesions. Most osteochondral lesions of the tibial plateau are localized in the medial and central regions and have a clearly traumatic etiopathogenesis [4].

In the ankle, the articular cartilage lesions recognize multiple causes; although there are idiopathic or non-traumatic forms, in most cases, these injuries have a traumatic origin and are mainly related to sports activity. An increase in their incidence is progressively occurring. The shear forces acting on the cartilage can produce superficial lesions without the involvement of the subchondral bone, while a direct high-energy trauma or repeated trauma (for example, in chronic instability) can damage the subchondral bone. According to the most recent literature reviews, osteochondral defects of the astragalus can occur in about 70% of ankle sprains and ankle fractures. From an epidemiological point of view, such lesions usually occur in young and active patients, 20-30 years of age, with high functional demands. Restoring the

damaged articular cartilage to a full and normal function condition has been difficult for orthopedic surgery.
Cartilage tissue, in fact, has limited healing potential and limited regenerative capacity. For this reason, joint damage can often become chronic and irreversible, giving rise to a chronic disability with a clinical picture characterized by deep pain, which worsens with the load and with physical activity. This progressive functional limitation is accompanied by widespread periarticular swelling and relapsing hydrarthrosis and with the possible development of early arthrosis.
Cartilage lesions can be classified according to the criteria of the ICRS (International Cartilage Repair Society) into full-thickness lesions or partial lesions depending on whether they extend deeply to expose the subchondral bone or not. Lesions of the articular cartilage that do not affect it at full thickness are incapable of spontaneous healing. In this type of injury, the subchondral bone represents a barrier between the cartilage lesion and the bone marrow-derived mesenchymal cells present in the subchondral spongy bone. In contrast, in full-thickness cartilage lesions, contact of the lesion with the mesenchymal cells of the subchondral spongy may occur. In this case, the process of spontaneous repair of cartilage damage produces fibrocartilaginous tissue that fills the injury site. Unfortunately, this tissue has lower mechanical characteristics than the hyaline articular cartilage and, over time, undergoes a progressive and inexorable degeneration. For this reason, the most significant efforts of scientific research are directed to attempts to fill the osteochondral lesion site with a tissue that possesses mechanical characteristics as similar as possible to those of the articular hyaline cartilage, and that is able to integrate biologically with the normal original articular cartilage, surrounding the site of injury. In this sense, the best results in minimally invasive arthroscopy repair of such lesions were obtained using bone marrow-derived mononuclear stem cells, scaffolds, and growth factors. Thanks to the technological advances of recent

years, the methods of regenerative surgery and orthobiology have rapidly progressed compared to the traditional transplantation of chondrocytes autologous, which required two separate interventions and had high costs. The transplantation of bone marrow mononucleate cells (MSC) has been achieved, an effective technique in repairing the lesion with hyaline cartilage through a single intervention, in combination with platelet gel or bioengineered scaffolds, capable of promoting the growth and differentiation of mesenchymal cells multipotent [5]. In the "one-step" method, instead of performing a preliminary phase of isolation and expansion of a certain line of mesenchymal cells, a transplant of the entire group of bone-marrow cells is performed. Thus, the bone marrow-derived stem cells are introduced into the joint together with all the other mononuclear cells and different growth factors present in the bone marrow blood and potentially endowed with a high regenerative stimulus. This procedure allows the collection and manipulation of cells inside the operating room, without the need for a preliminary phase to be performed in the laboratory.

Mesenchymal stem cells reside in specialized microenvironments called niches. The niche is fundamental to support the function of MSCs and to maintain a correct balance between self-renewal and progression towards a differentiative line. Bone marrow tissue is a complex microenvironment comprising endothelial cells and structures (including sinusoidal, arterial and transitional microvascular capillaries) and mesenchymal stromal cells (including mesenchymal stem cells and progenitor line cells, as well as precursor cell elements of the osteogenic line, chondrocytes, and adipocytes) [6]. MSCs can replace cells that undergo necrosis and apoptosis and support the cell rambling of various tissues in young adults. In case of severe tissue damage, MSCs may be attracted to chemotaxis at the site of injury, where they release biologically active factors that stimulate the processes of damage repair and tissue regeneration. MSCs can be taken from the bone marrow blood and conveyed to the injury site or can be expanded in the laboratory and administered later to the patient, either systemically or by local inoculation. Conveyed at the injury site, these cells produce biological factors that inhibit fibrous-scarring tissue formation and apoptosis, promote neoangiogenesis, and stimulate multipotent cell lines residing in the lesion site tissue to replicate and differentiate into regenerative tissue units. Mesenchymal cells of bone-marrow origin have historically been the first stem cells to be identified, and the ease of collection and the relatively high amount of locally present MSCs make bone marrow tissue still a commonly used source of mesenchymal stem cells. MSCs can be used as an expanded cell suspension in culture or as a simple concentrate of bone marrow tissue. Advances in regenerative medicine have shown that mesenchymal stem cells are able to replicate and regenerate both bone and cartilage tissue without the need for prior manipulation in the laboratory.

Surgical technique

The patient is positioned in prone decubitus under spinal or general anesthesia. We proceed with the preparation of the sterile field and the heparinization of surgical instruments. We proceed with the identification of the upper arch of the posterior iliac crest homolateral to the lesion. Through a trocar, 60 ml of bone marrow blood is taken and centrifuged with a special dedicated device for 12 minutes. The bone marrow concentrate is suctioned with a sterile syringe at the end of the process. The patient is then placed supine with ischemic lace at the root of the lower limb. Standard anteromedial and anterolateral arthroscopic accesses to the tibiotarsal or knee are created. The lesion is found and evaluated. The lesion is cleared up to expose a bed of healthy and well-vascularized subchondral spongy bone, free of sclerosis. With special instruments, the preparation of hyaluronic acid scaffolds and midollar mononuclear cells is placed under direct arthroscopic control to obtain the maximum possible coverage of the lesion. Finally, the area is covered with fibrin glue. Repeated movements of the joint subjected to a procedure are performed to check the stability of the implant and the absence of impingement with the joint structures. Finally, the arthroscopic accesses are sutured [2,7]. There may be a need, in OC ankle lesions, to perform an arthrotomic access (medial or lateral), rarely preceded by a malleolar osteotomy, to better expose the site of the lesion on the talar dome.

Indications and clinical results

The use of the bone marrow concentrate is indicated in osteochondral lesions of the femoral condyles (figg.1,2) and of the femoral-patellar joint and in the treatment of dissecting osteochondrites [2]: regenerative medicine, compared to the reparative medicine widely used in the management of small lesions (< 1 cm^2), has become indispensable for the larger (> 1 cm^2) and deeper (> 0.5 cm) ones. For this reason, where the in-

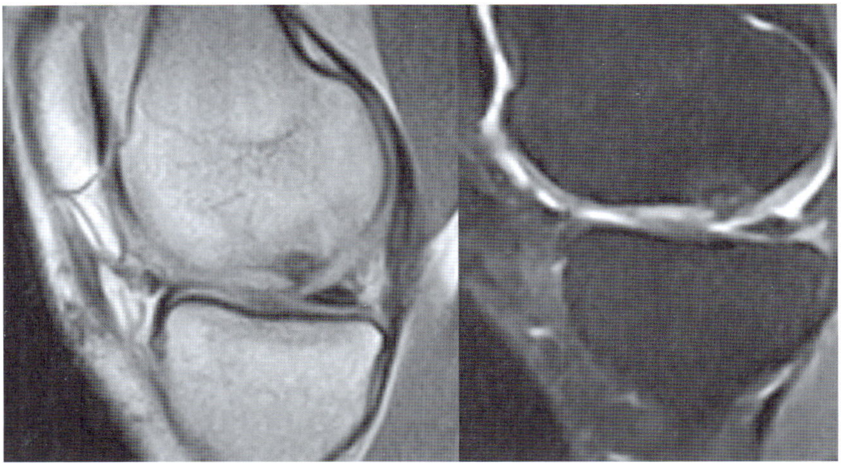

Figure 1 Male patient, 28 years old. Osteochondral lesion femoral condyle, pre-operative MRI

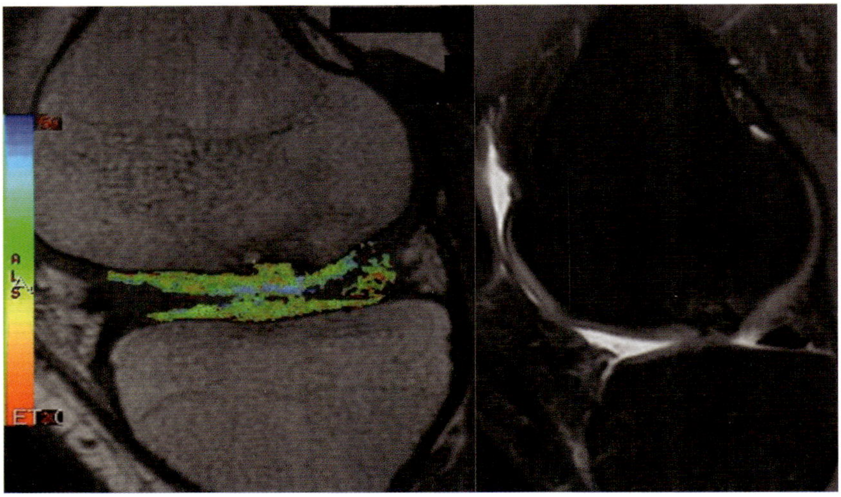

Figure 2 Follow-up at 2 years, IKDC 95 points, RMN control with T2-mapping sequence

volvement of the subchondral bone is present (ankle), the filling of the lesion will have to make use of "orthobiological" techniques, and numerous studies have proven this, demonstrating the safety and effectiveness of the "one-step" procedure [8,9]. In 2016 Buda et al. [10] demonstrated a significant improvement in the AOFAS score in a series of 56 consecutive patients at 2 and 3 years of follow-up, with a result inversely related to the presence of radiographic signs of a significant arthritic degeneration of the ankle at the time of surgery; implant stability was evaluated with an MRI, which showed a complete peripheral integration of the regenerated tissue with a highly homogeneous surface appearance (fig. 3). Similarly, for the treatment of OC lesions of the tibial plafond, the same outcomes were highlighted in a 2018 study [11], observing only in 5 patients a hypertrophy of the regenerated tissue (3) and an incomplete repair of the lesion (2). Therefore the results in the treatment of OC lesions have shown that the use of mesenchymal cells of bone marrow origin can be a

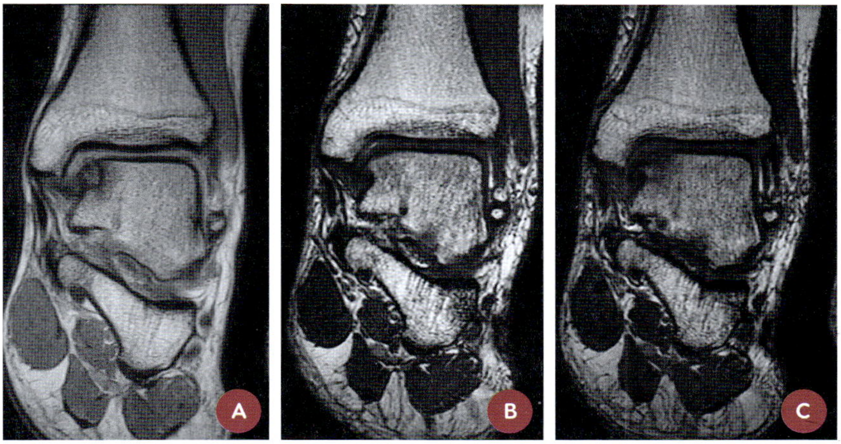

Figure 3 (A) Male patient, 23 years old, osteochondral lesion of the astragalus, pre-operative MRI; B) Clinical control (AOFAS 90 points) and imaging at 6 months; C) Follow-up to 1 year with RMN, AOFAS 100 points

valid support for the orthopedic surgeon; In particular, the bone marrow concentrate taken from the iliac crest contains an adequate amount of progenitor cells and growth factors which, associated with biocompatible scaffolds and a mini-invasive technique, allows to achieve optimal clinical and functional objectives in the medium-long term for the patient suffering from osteochondral lesions.

References

1. Aurich M, Hofmann GO, Rolauffs B, et al. Differences in injury pattern and prevalence of cartilage lesions in knee and ankle joints: a retrospective cohort study. Orthop Rev 2014;6:5611.
2. Buda R, Vannini F, Cavallo M, et al. Osteochondral lesions of the knee: a new one-step repair technique with bonemarrow- derived cells. J Bone Joint Surg Am 2010;92(Suppl 2):2-11.
3. O'Loughlin PF, Heyworth BE, Kennedy JG. Current concepts in the diagnosis and treatment of osteochondral lesions of the ankle. Am J Sports Med 2010;38:392-404.
4. Elias I, Raikin SM, Schweitzer ME, et al. Osteochondral lesions of the distal tibial plafond: localization and morphologic characteristics with an anatomical grid. Foot Ankle Int 2009;30:524-9.
5. Meirelles Lda S, Fontes AM, Covas DT, et al. Mechanisms involved in the therapeutic properties of mesenchymal stem cells.

Cytokine Growth Factor Rev 2009;20(5-6):419-27.
6. Pintus E, Baldassarri M, Perazzo L, et al. Stem cells in osteochondral tissue engineering. Adv Exp Med Biol 2018;1058:359-72. doi: 10.1007/978-3-319-76711-6_16.
7. Giannini S, Buda R, Vannini F, et al. One-step bone marrowderived cell transplantation in talar osteochondral lesions. Clin Orthop Relat Res 2009;467:3307-20.
8. Giannini S, Buda R, Cavallo M, et al. Cartilage repair evolution in post-traumatic osteochondral lesions of the talus: from open field autologous chondrocyte to bone-marrow-derived cells transplantation. Injury 2010;41:1196-1203.
9. Giannini S, Buda R, Battaglia M, et al. One-step repair in talar osteochondral lesions: 4-year clinical results and t2- map ping capability in outcome prediction. Am J Sports Med 2013;41:511-8.
10. Buda R, Castagnini F, Cavallo M, et al. One-step bone marrow-derived cells transplantation and joint debridement for osteochondral lesions of the talus in ankle osteoarthritis: clinical and radiological outcomes at 36 months. Arch Orthop Trauma Surg 2016;136:107-16.
11. Baldassarri M, Perazzo L, Ricciarelli M, et al. Regenerative treatment of osteochondral lesions of distal tibial plafond. Eur J Orthop Surg Traumatol 2018;28:1199-1207. doi: 10.1007/ s00590-018-2161-7. Epub 2018 Feb 23.

CHAPTER 2

BIOPHYSICAL STIMULATION IN REGENERATIVE MEDICINE

Simona Salati[1], Stefania Setti[2], Ruggero Cadossi[3], Matteo Cadossi[4]

1) Research coordinator, Igea Clinical Biophysics, Carpi (MO)

2) Project leader Orthopaedics, Igea Clinical Biophysics, Carpi (MO)

3) President, Igea Clinical Biophysics, Carpi (MO)

4) Vice president, Igea Clinical Biophysics, Carpi (MO)

Introduction

The articular surfaces of the bone are covered with cartilage that favors the movement of the articular heads and absorb the mechanical stresses to which the joint is subjected. Articular cartilage is a hypocellular tissue, poorly vascularized, composed of a dense matrix of collagen and proteoglycans. This complex structure allows articular cartilage to perform its biomechanical role by providing low friction and a highly wear-resistant surface to both tangential stress and compression [1].

On the other hand, the hypocellular and avascular nature of the cartilage gives this tissue poor regenerative abilities, insufficient to repair the damage induced by trauma or the catabolic effects of inflammatory reactions resulting from them. If these lesions are not treated, they often progress to tissue degeneration: the cartilage progressively thins and tears, the subchondral bone tissue is progressively exposed until a picture of osteoarthritis (OA) is established [2]. The most advanced treatments for inflammatory and degenerative cartilage diseases aim to accelerate the repair of cartilage tissue and rebuild the functional properties of damaged tissues [3]. Several strategies are currently proposed for cartilage repair, including chondro-abrasion, microfractures, or techniques aimed at filling cartilage damage with autologous chondrocytes grown ex vivo, mesenchymal stem cells (MSCSs) isolated from the bone marrow (BM), or osteochondral grafts [4]. So far, these treatments have not offered reproducible and stable substitutions over time. More specifically, surgical procedures cannot replicate the biological composition and biomechanical characteristics of native cartilage, which determines the formation of fibrous tissue with lower mechanical properties and limited duration in time.

For this reason, patients often continue to report persistent symptoms such as pain and intra-articular effusion. In addition, the joint environment is severely modified after a surgical procedure, even if minimally invasive such as arthroscopy. In particular, the concentration of pro-inflammatory cytokines and inflammatory cells in the synovial fluid increases significantly, leading to degradation of the extracellular matrix and loss of proteoglycans. During the inflammatory response, the physiological maintenance of cartilage is lost, guaranteed by the balance between anabolic and catabolic activities. Because of its low reparative capacity, it is of fundamental importance to maintain the health of the articular cartilage in all its components, cells, extracellular matrix, and subchondral bone. This can be achieved by stimulating chondrocyte activity and inhibiting the damage caused by inflammation. To this end, the concept of chondroprotection identifies different pharmacological, physical, or surgical treatments, used both individually and in combination, which promote the preservation of the cartilage itself or aim to limit damage due to degenerative, pathological, inflammatory, or traumatic causes.

The scientific literature has amply demonstrated that biophysical stimulation is able to perform a protective action on joint tissues. Moreover, recent observations have highlighted the ability of biophysical stimulation to act by stimulating the synthesis of engineered tissue in vitro starting from autologous chondrocytes of the patient or MSCs. Based on these observations, a dual action of biophysical stimulation in tissue engineering strategies can be hypothesized. In vitro, biophysical stimulation promotes cell proliferation, chondrocyte differentiation, scaffold colonization, and extracellular matrix synthesis (ECM), thus favoring the formation of a 3D engineered tissue with structural and functional properties that better reproduce the characteristics of native cartilage. Biophysical stimulation protects the engineered construct from the catabolic activity of pro-inflammatory cytokines in the clinic, favoring a better integration of the construct at the implant site.

Biophysical stimulation: mechanism of action

Biophysical stimulation consists in the application of non-ionizing physical stimuli, such as pulsed electromagnetic fields (PEMFs), for therapeutic purposes. PEMFs are currently successfully used in the orthopedic field as a safe and non-invasive treatment to accelerate the healing of fractures and promote joint cartilage repair.

Physiologically, the human body controls inflammation through the activation of numerous signal pathways, such as signal pathways mediated by adenosine receptors, in particular subtypes A_{2A} and A_3 [5,6]. In 2002, the research group coordinated by Prof. Varani showed that EMPs interact with adenosine receptors. In human neutrophils, stimulation with CEMP exerts a strong adenosine-agonist effect specific to A_{2A} and A_3 [7,8] receptors. This effect, mediated by the increase in the number of receptors in the membrane, determines a significant increase in intracellular cyclic AMP (cAMP) and a reduction in the release of the superoxide anion (O2-), suggesting an anti-inflammatory effect. This action mechanism was subsequently confirmed in human chondrocytes and synoviocytes [9]. In the same period, Cohen described the role of the A_{2A} receptor in regulating joint tissue inflammation: in an animal model of septic osteoarthritis, Cohen showed that the A_{2A} receptor-specific agonist, ATL 146e, is able to reduce cartilage damage significantly, synovial inflammation, and infiltration of leukocytes [10]. On these bases, the role of pulsed electromagnetic fields in the protection of cartilage tissue and the regulation of inflammation in the joint environment has been hypothesized.

Effect of pulsed electromagnetic fields on in vitro engineered construct

Anabolic effect

The scientific literature agrees that pulsed electromagnetic fields influence chondrocytes maintained under different experimental conditions (cell cultures, cartilage explants, and 3D constructs) by increasing cell proliferation and synthesis of CME components, such as proteoglycans (PG) and type II collagen. Exposure to PEMFs increases the incorporation of H3-thymidine into human articular chondrocytes in vitro [11]. In addition, pulsed electromagnetic fields are able to stimulate anabolic activities, such as proteoglycan synthesis, in ex vivo [12] cartilage explants. In particular, De Mattei showed that the increase in PGs synthesis induced by biophysical stimulation in human cartilage explants is of the same magnitude as that induced by the main anabolic cartilage growth factor insulin-like growth factor (IGF-1) [13].

Anti-inflammatory effect

Numerous experimental evidences show that stimulation of A_{2A} or A_3 receptors mediates inhibition of the signal pathway of NF-Kb [14,15]. In chondrocytes and synoviocytes, NF-kB regulates the expression of cyclooxygenase type 2 (COX-2), metalloproteinases (MMPs), and numerous genes involved in inflammatory response [16]. Activation of A_{2A} and A_3 receptors in the presence of PEMFs reduces the release of prostaglandin E2 (PGE2) and the expression of COX-2 in bovine synoviocytes, thus reducing inflammation and subsequent degradation of cartilage [17]. In particular, PEMF stimulation of A_{2A} and A_3 receptors in human synoviocytes inhibits the MAPK p38 and NF-kB pathways, thus leading to a reduction in the synthesis of TNF-α, IL-1β, and other mediators involved in joint inflammation [18].

In human synovial fibroblasts taken from patients with osteoarthritis, Ongaro has shown that PEMF stimulation reduces the synthesis of inflammatory mediators such as PGE2 and pro-inflammatory cytokines (IL-6 and IL-8) while stimulating the release of anti-inflammatory cytokines, such as interleukin-10 (IL-10) [19]. Finally, the same authors showed that pulsed electromagnetic fields are able to counteract the inhibition of chondrogenesis induced by pro-inflammatory cytokines (such as IL-1 β) in mesenchymal stem cells by suggesting the use of biophysical stimulation as a therapeutic strategy to improve the clinical outcome of cartilage repair procedures [20].

Chondrogenic effect in mesenchymal stem cells

The scientific literature reports numerous experimental evidence that shows how pulsed electromagnetic fields are able to enhance the paracrine and reparative functions of mesenchymal stem cells. MSCs support chondrogenic differentiation and represent a promising cellular source for tissue engineering. Despite these high potentials, neocartilage generated by conventional repair methods based on MSCs commonly contains a mixture of fibro-cartilage and hyaline cartilage that does not achieve the mechanical and functional properties of native cartilage. For this reason, numerous efforts have been made in the medical-scientific community in order to improve the quality and functionality of the regenerated tissue. Among the potential mechanisms for modulation of chondrogenic differentiation and functionality of mesenchymal stem cells, stimulation through PEMFs has been identified.

Several studies have analyzed the effects of PEMFs treatment on the chondrocyte differentiation of mesenchymal stem cells derived from bone marrow, adipose tissue, umbilical cord, synovial fluid, and peripheral blood. The results, however, are partly discordant. Some studies report modest improvements in gene expression of Sox9, aggrecan, collagen type II (Col 2), and GAG deposition, while other studies show mild effects to no effects. These divergences are related to significant differences in stimulation protocols with PEMFs. Parate characterized the effects of pulsed electromagnetic fields exposure on the chondrocyte differentiation of MSCs as the field amplitude, duration of exposure, and dosage [21] vary. The authors demonstrate that short, single exposures to low-amplitude pulsed electromagnetic fields (2 mTesla, mT) effectively stimulate chondrogenesis. Exposure to PEMFs in the early stages of chondrogenic differentiation of mesenchymal stem cells induces an increase in intracellular $Ca2+$ concentrations that are optimal for promoting chondrogenesis initiation. In particular, the authors demonstrate the involvement of mechanosensitive TRP channels, TRPC1 and

TRPV4, in chondrogenic differentiation stimulated by exposure to pulsed electromagnetic fields.

Initially, the potential application of mesenchymal stem cells for cartilage repair was postulated on the basis of their ability to differentiate to chondrocytes, and it has subsequently become increasingly evident that part of the reparative capacity of MSCs is attributable to their paracrine activity. In non-contact co-culture systems between MSCs and primary chondrocytes, trophic factors released by MSCs were responsible for increasing chondrocyte proliferation, maintaining the differentiated phenotype, and synthesizing ECM 22 components. The paracrine action of mesenchymal stem cells is further supported by preclinical studies showing that intra-articular injection of MSCs prevents the development of post-traumatic arthritis and promotes cartilage regeneration in damaged articles [23]. Recently, Parate has shown that the pro-chondrogenic effect induced by exposure to PEMFs can be primarily attributed to their modulation of the secretome of mesenchymal stem cells [24]. In this work, the authors demonstrate that PEMFs stimulation is able to modulate the chondrogenic, chemotactic, anti-inflammatory, and anti-apoptotic activities of the secretome of mesenchymal stem cells. In addition, this work highlights the importance of optimizing pulsed electromagnetic fields exposure parameters for MSCS subjected to different culture conditions: MSCS grown in 2D or 3D show distinct sensitivities to stimulation with pulsed electromagnetic fields, responding more favorably to amplitudes of 3mT and 2 mT, respectively.

In this perspective, stimulation with PEMFs, through its effects on the paracrine activity of mesenchymal stem cells, represents a valid treatment to promote the regeneration of damaged cartilage within a pro-inflammatory joint environment.

Effect of pulsed electromagnetic fields on in vivo engineered construct

If, on the one hand, the stimulation with PEMFs is able to improve the characteristics of the engineered tissue in vitro, on the other hand, it favors a better integration of the construct in the implantation site and, through the control of the articular microenvironment, prevents the catabolic effects induced by inflammation.

The chondroprotective activity of pulsed electromagnetic fields was first described by Ciombor et al. [25] in a model of spontaneous osteoarthritis in Hartley guinea pigs. The authors showed that exposure to pulsed electromagnetic fields counteracts cartilage degeneration as measured by Mankin score. In particular, PEMFs stimulation induces a significant reduction in the levels of pro-inflammatory cytokine IL-1β coupled with an increase in the levels of Transforming Growth Factor-1 beta (TGF-1β). This growth factor stimulates the synthesis of type II collagen and counteracts the production of pro-inflammatory cytokines. More recently, the research group coordinated by Dr. Fini has shown that pulsed electromagnetic fields are able to stop the progression of osteoarthritis, limit surface fissures and cartilage fibrillation, preserve the thickness of cartilage tissue, and prevent sclerosis of the subchondral bone in guinea pigs Dunkin Hartley [26,27].

In the context of tissue engineering, these results support the use of PEMFs in order to exert a protective effect on the engineered construct after its implantation. In an animal model of autologous osteochondral grafts, pulsed electromagnetic fields have been shown to promote graft integration and prevent resorption 28. In addition, in the synovial fluid of animals treated with PEMFs, the authors measured significantly lower levels of pro-inflammatory cytokines, such as IL-1β and TNF-α, and a higher concentration of TGF-β1 re-treated animals, indicative of a more favorable joint environment [28]. Subsequently, these results were confirmed in studies conducted in rabbit osteochondral lesions treated with collagen scaffold seeded with bone marrow cell concentrate (BMC). Combined treatment with BMC and PEMFs demonstrated a better ability to osteochondral regeneration than treatments applied individually. The authors reported a significant improvement in the quality of regenerated cartilage and subchondral bone [29] (fig. 1).

Recently, Hung's research group at Columbia University investigated the effect of pulsed electromagnetic fields on the structural and functional quality of engineered osteochondral constructs and the post-implantation joint environment in a model of focal cartilage lesions in dog [30]. The results demonstrate that stimulation with PEMFs increases cell content, extracellular matrix deposition, and integration of engineered constructs in vitro. In vivo, stimulation with PEMFs, performed after implantation of engineered cartilage grafts, promotes the formation of a uniform repair

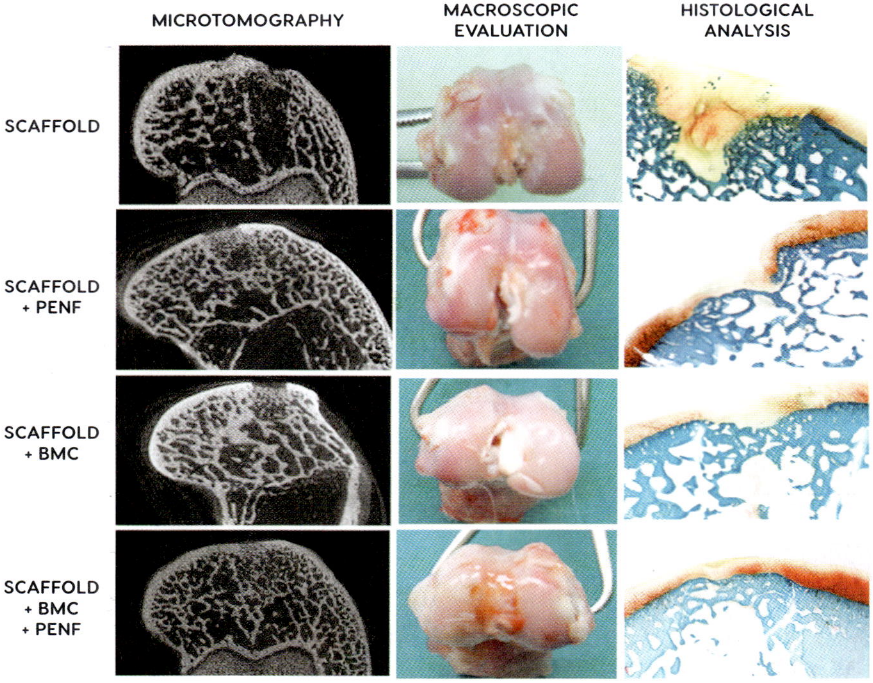

Figure 1 Microtomography, macroscopic evaluation, and histological analysis of osteochondral lesions treated with scaffold, scaffold + PEMFs, scaffold + BMC, and scaffold + BMC + PEMFs.

tissue and reduces levels of pro-inflammatory cytokines in the joint environment (fig. 2).
Overall, these results suggest that stimulation with PEMFs represents a non-invasive clinical outcome that improves the properties of pre-implantation cartilage and reduces inflammatory catabolic activities in the post-implantation, thus favoring the achievement of positive and stable clinical results in the long term.

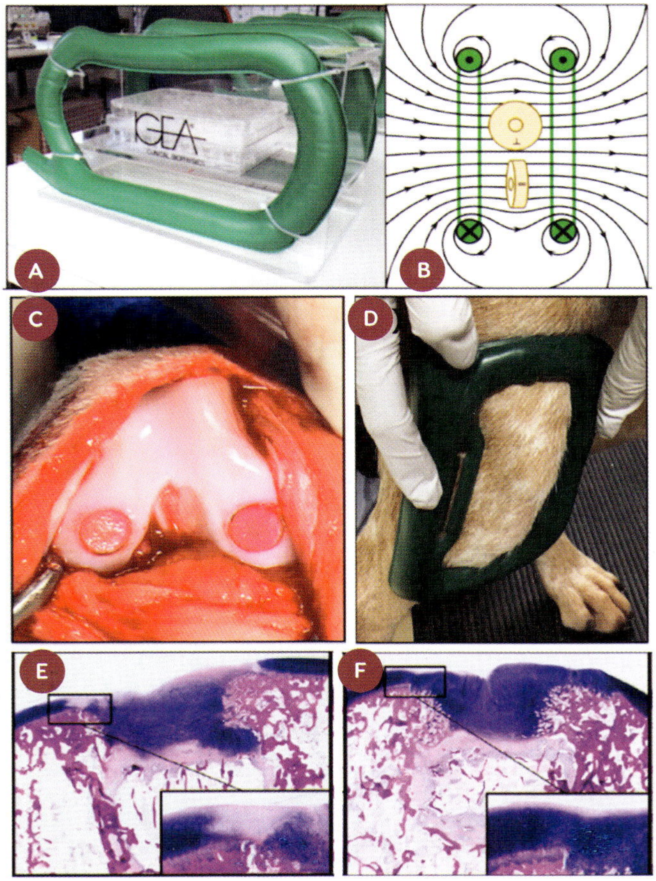

Figure 2 a) In vitro EMF Exposure System; b) Magnetic field lines with engineered constructs arranged in perpendicular (⊥) or parallel (=) orientation to the magnetic field; c) engineered osteochondral grafts implanted in femoral condyles; d) Solenoid used for in vivo study; hematoxylin-eosin staining of histologies representative of the engineered construct not stimulated (e) and stimulated with PEMFs (f).

Clinical study

The effect of biophysical stimulation in association with tissue engineering techniques was evaluated in a randomized controlled clinical trial performed at the Rizzoli Orthopaedic Institute.
In this study, biophysical stimulation was associated with the surgical treatment of osteochondral lesions of the astragalus by transplanting Bone Marrow Aspirate Concentrate (BMAC) on collagen scaffolds in a single operating session (one-step).

Methods

The study was approved by the Institute's Ethics Committee. The inclusion criteria were as follows: patients with post-traumatic or degenerative astragalus osteochondral lesions of grade III and IV according to the Outerbridge classification; ages between 18 and 50 years; patients with lesions evaluated by MRI and candidates for transplantation with autologous bone marrow mononuclear cells (MNCs) in arthroscopy. The exclusion criteria were as follows: patients who had previously undergone other ankle surgeries, carriers of an articular prosthesis in the lower extremities, patients suffering from rheumatoid arthritis, autoimmune diseases, systemic pathologies, malignant neoplasms, and with a BMI >30 Kg/m2.
Patients underwent autologous MNCs on a scaffold by one-step technique. The bone marrow was collected in sterility from the patient's posterior iliac crest under prone decubitus and general or spinal anesthesia. Considering that only the first 2 ml of aspirate contains a significant amount of MSCS, a specific procedure [31] has been adopted to optimize the collection. The collected bone marrow was processed directly in the operating room using a device for the separation and concentration of mononuclear cells from bone marrow blood. From 60 mL of bone marrow aspirate, 6 mL of buffy coat was obtained, containing MSCs and other populations of nucleated cells that make up the bone marrow microenvironment.
After this first phase, with the patient in supine decubitus, arthroscopy of the

ankle was performed through the standard procedure with anteromedial and anterolateral access. The lesion was identified, the detached cartilage fragment was removed, and the lesion was cleaned up to the healthy subchondral bone. The collagen scaffold was sown with about 2 mL of bone marrow concentrate and subsequently placed on the lesion. 1 mL of fibrin-rich plasma (PRF), obtained from autologous venous blood the day before surgery, was sown on the scaffold after its placement at the site of the injury. After the surgery, all patients underwent the same rehabilitation protocol: active and passive early mobilization of the ankle without load for 6 weeks, followed by 4 weeks of partial load and finally full load on the operated limb. Patients in the experimental group were stimulated with PEMFs (I-ONE Terapia, IGEA S.p.A. Carpi, Italy) with a peak magnetic field intensity of 1.5 mT and a frequency of 75 Hz, 4 hours a day for 60 days starting from the 3rd day after surgery.

Joint function and pain were assessed using: Visual Analog Scale (VAS), 36-Item Short Form Survey (SF-36), American Orthopedic Foot and Ankle Society (AOFAS) score ed EuroQoL pre-surgery and respectively 1, 2, 6, and 12 months after surgery.

The minimum difference in the AOFAS score that has been considered clinically relevant is at least 10 points. On this basis, the statistical power of the sample was calculated on the assumption that the AOFAS score at 12 months was greater than 12 units in the experimental group. Considering an alpha value of 0.05 and a statistical power of 80%, the estimated sample size for each group was 13 units. Considering a dropout rate of about 10%, the sample size was 15 units per group.

Results

From September 2012 to December 2012, 30 patients (22 males and 8 females) with an average age of 38.2 years were enrolled in the study. Patients were assigned to the experimental or control group before surgery by randomization with a sealed envelope technique.

Patient characteristics did not differ between 2 groups at the time of enrollment, with the exception of the SF-36 score, which was significantly higher in the experimental group.

No major complications occurred, and all patients were discharged within 2 days of surgery. During the first 2 months after surgery, patients in the investigational group used I-ONE Therapy (fig. 3) for an average of 4.2 ± 2.0 hours per day.

Clinical improvement was observed in both groups from enrollment to the last follow-up at 12 months. In the control group, the AOFAS score improved from 48.9 ± 23.0 points in the pre-operative period to 79.9 ± 16.8 and 81.0 ± 20.2 points at 6 and 12 months of follow-up, respectively ($p = 0.003$ and $p = 0.002$ compared to baseline). In the experimental group, the AOFAS score improved from 54.1 ± 20.1 pre-operative to 88.9 ± 6.7 and 94.3 ± 7 to 6 and 12 months of follow-up, respectively ($p < 0.0001$ and $p < .0001$ compared to baseline) (Figure 4a). The AOFAS score

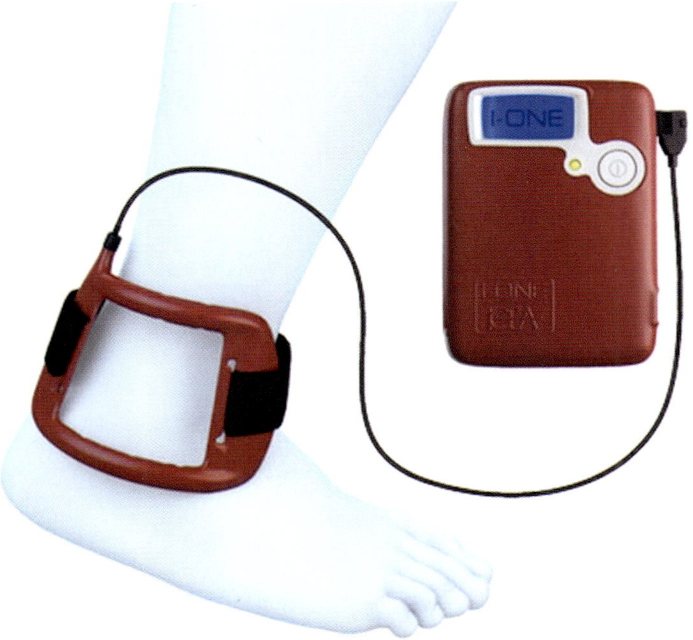

Figure 3 Medical device for PEMFs stimulation, I-ONE Therapy.

in the experimental group was significantly higher than in the control group at 6 months (p = 0.035) and 12 months (p = 0.014) after intervention [32].

In both groups at 30 days, a significant improvement in pain evaluated by VAS was observed; however, this improvement was maintained overtime only in patients treated with I-ONE Therapy. In the control group, a tendency to worsen over time was observed. Patients in the experimental group report pain significantly less than 2 (p = 0.039), 6 (p = 0.024) and 12 months (p = 0.040) of follow-up compared to controls (Figure 4b)

In addition, during the first 30 days, SF-36 decreased significantly in both groups compared to baseline due to postoperative pain and absence of load during rehabilitation. At 6 and 12 months of follow-up, a significant improvement in SF-36 was observed in patients treated with I-ONE Terapia compared to controls (p = 0.004 and P < .0001, respectively).

These results confirm the positive effect of biophysical stimulation in a clinical context of tissue engineering, showing significantly better functional results in the group of stimulated patients than in controls. Interestingly, the AOFAS score of patients treated with I-ONE Terapia is not only higher than in controls but also has limited

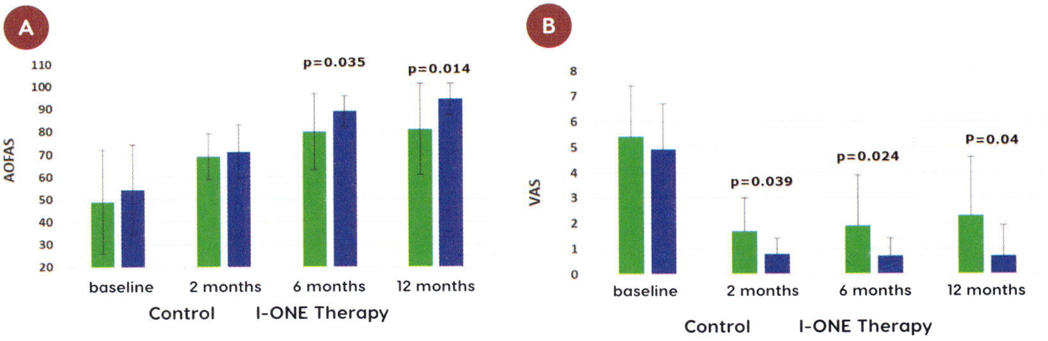

Figure 4 Mean AOFAS scores in the experimental (I-ONE Therapy) and control (a) group, mean VAS values in the experimental group (I-ONE Therapy), and control (b). The values are reported as an average ± SD.

standard variation at 12 months. This data indicates a greater homogeneity of the results with AOFAS score values close to the average value suggesting a frequently positive clinical result for patients stimulated with I-ONE Terapia. On the contrary, a significant standard deviation of the AOFAS score at 12 months is observed in the control group. This figure is indicative of a large prognostic variability, with clinical results on average less satisfactory.

Similar results have also been reported in patients with osteochondral knee lesions treated with autologous matrix-assisted chondrocyte implantation (MACI) [33].

The authors report significantly better clinical outcomes (as measured by the International Knee Documentation Committee- IKDC score) in patients treated with I-ONE Therapy than controls at 5 years of follow-up ($p = 0.001$). In addition, the I-ONE Therapy group achieves significantly better resolution from pain (follow-up of 2 and 60 months) than controls.

In contrast to these works, Reilingh recently published the results of a randomized clinical trial aimed at evaluating the effect of biophysical stimulation on the return to sports activity in patients suffering from osteochondral lesions of astragalus treated with arthroscopic debridement and microfractures. The authors report that the percentage of patients who resume sports activity and the median time to resume activity do not differ significantly between the stimulated and control groups. Similarly, the authors do not show significant differences between the groups regarding the study's secondary endpoints (such as functional results and computed tomography results) [34].

A careful analysis of the results shows that 96% of patients returned to sport within the 30th week of surgery in the group treated with I-ONE Therapy. In contrast, the same percentage was reached in the control group at the 52nd week after surgery [35]. In addition, according to the information provided in the article published by Reilingh, 25% of patients used the device less than 180 hours (3 hours/day). Numerous clinical studies have shown that average daily stimulation has a signi-

ficant impact on treatment outcome, so 25% of patients who have not completed therapy may have adversely affected the results of this study.
The scientific literature generally agrees that biophysical stimulation can be successfully used in association with tissue engineering approaches for cartilage repair. By promoting the anabolic activity of implanted cells and peri-articular tissues and protecting the construct from the catabolic effects of inflammation, biophysical stimulation promotes the achievement of positive and lasting clinical results.

Discussion

The importance of different regenerative medicine techniques associated with classic surgical approaches is now universally recognized. However, the clinical results of tissue engineering for cartilage repair are highly variable and sometimes conflicting. The existence of patient-specific factors and lesion-specific factors that significantly influence the clinical outcome after tissue engineering approaches for the treatment of osteochondral lesions [36] has been described.
From a clinical point of view, the formation of fibrous tissue with lower functional and mechanical properties than native cartilage and difficulties in integrating the engineered constructure with the surrounding environment and with the subchondral bone have been reported.
Several authors emphasize the need to improve the quality of engineered tissue to improve the clinical outcome of regenerative medicine approaches in treating osteochondral defects.
From this point of view, the transplantation of bone marrow mononucleate cells, enriched in MSCs, indeed represents a step forward in the attempt to replace the damaged cartilage tissue with a functional tissue similar to native cartilage. However, even this approach has some limitations. Despite the ability of mesenchymal stem cells to differentiate in a chondrogenic sense, the final differentiation more resembles the phenotype associated with endochondral ossification rather

than articular chondrocytes [37]. Recent studies have shown that the intrinsic chondrogenic differentiation program of MSCs gives rise to a hypertrophic phenotype similar to the early physiological phases of the endochondral ossification process, thus resulting in the production of fibrocartilage and hypertrophic tissues [38]. On this basis, the hypocellularity of cartilage and the lack of nutrient supply, combined with the inefficient production of an ECM typical of hyaline cartilage, generates a tissue unable to activate a functional healing response, thus limiting the usefulness of mesenchymal stem cells in the cartilage repair [39].

Several elements can compromise the success of a regenerative medicine procedure; however, local inflammation is probably the most critical condition in tissue engineering. Therefore, the local microenvironment of the treated joint should be considered the most important variable that affects the success of regenerative therapy: it has a substantial impact on in situ degradation and survival of engineered constructs.

The surgical procedure required to implant the engineered cartilage triggers an inflammatory response, which represents a potentially harmful event for the articular cartilage and the engineered construct, which could eventually compromise the positive effects expected from regenerative medicine. The results of preclinical research and clinical trials suggest that pulsed electromagnetic fields may play a key role in the success of tissue engineering approaches, exerting a positive effect in both in vitro and clinical phases of tissue engineering.

In the in vitro phase, exposure to PEMFs stimulates chondrocyte differentiation of mesenchymal stem cells [21], the proliferation of chondrocytes [11], and extracellular matrix deposition [12,13].

In the presence of scaffolds, stimulation with PEMFs ensures better functional properties and better integration of the engineered construct [30].

In the clinical phase, the use of mesenchymal stem cells after surgical implantation of the construct controls joint inflammation [28.30], protects against the catabolic effect of inflammatory cytokines [20], and stimulates the anabolic action of both the transplanted cells and the surrounding cartilage [29].

References

1. Ulrich-Vinther M, Maloney MD, Schwarz EM, Rosier R, O'Keefe RJ. Articular Cartilage Biology: J Am Acad Orthop Surg. 2003;11(6):421-430. doi:10.5435/00124635-200311000-00006
2. Holland TA, Tessmar JKV, Tabata Y, Mikos AG. Transforming growth factor-β1 release from oligo(poly(ethylene glycol) fumarate) hydrogels in conditions that model the cartilage wound healing environment. J Controlled Release. 2004;94(1):101-114. doi:10.1016/j.jconrel.2003.09.007
3. CITER (Cardiff Institute of Tissue Engineering and Repair), Cardiff School of Biosciences, Museum Avenue, Cardiff, CF10 3US, Wales, UK, Redman S, Oldfield S, Archer C. Current strategies for articular cartilage repair. Eur Cell Mater. 2005;9:23-32. doi:10.22203/eCM.v009a04
4. Ahmed TAE, Hincke MT. Strategies for Articular Cartilage Lesion Repair and Functional Restoration. Tissue Eng Part B Rev. 2010;16(3):305-329. doi:10.1089/ten.teb.2009.0590
5. Tesch AM, MacDonald MH, Kollias-Baker C, Benton HP. Chondrocytes respond to adenosine via A2receptors and activity is potentiated by an adenosine deaminase inhibitor and a phosphodiesterase inhibitor. Osteoarthritis Cartilage. 2002;10(1):34-43. doi:10.1053/joca.2001.0479
6. Borea PA, Gessi S, Bar-Yehuda S, Fishman P. A3 Adenosine Receptor: Pharmacology and Role in Disease. In: Wilson CN, Mustafa SJ, eds. Adenosine Receptors in Health and Disease. Vol 193. Springer Berlin Heidelberg; 2009:297-327. doi:10.1007/978-3-540-89615-9_10
7. Varani K, Gessi S, Merighi S, et al. Effect of low-frequency electromagnetic fields on A 2A adenosine receptors in human neutrophils. Br J Pharmacol. 2002;136(1):57-66. doi:10.1038/sj.bjp.0704695
8. Varani K, Gessi S, Merighi S, et al. Alteration of A3 adenosine receptors in human neutrophils and low frequency electromagnetic fields. Biochem Pharmacol. 2003;66(10):1897-1906. doi:10.1016/S0006-2952(03)00454-4
9. Varani K, De Mattei M, Vincenzi F, et al. Characterization of adenosine receptors in bovine chondrocytes and fibroblast-like synoviocytes exposed to low frequency low energy pulsed electromagnetic fields. Osteoarthritis Cartilage. 2008;16(3):292-304. doi:10.1016/j.joca.2007.07.004
10. Cohen SB, Gill SS, Baer GS, Leo BM, Scheld WM, Diduch DR. Reducing joint destruction due to septic arthrosis using an adenosine2A receptor agonist. J Orthop Res. 2004;22(2):427-435. doi:10.1016/j.orthres.2003.08.011

11. Pezzetti F, De Mattei M, Caruso A, et al. Effects of pulsed electromagnetic fields on human chondrocytes: an in vitro study. Calcif Tissue Int. 1999;65(5):396-401.
12. De Mattei M, Pasello M, Pellati A, et al. Effects of electromagnetic fields on proteoglycan metabolism of bovine articular cartilage explants. Connect Tissue Res. 2003;44(3-4):154-159.
13. De Mattei M, Pellati A, Pasello M, et al. Effects of physical stimulation with electromagnetic field and insulin growth factor-I treatment on proteoglycan synthesis of bovine articular cartilage. Osteoarthritis Cartilage. 2004;12(10):793-800. doi:10.1016/j.joca.2004.06.012
14. Lee JY, Jhun BS, Oh YT, et al. Activation of adenosine A3 receptor suppresses lipopolysaccharide-induced TNF-alpha production through inhibition of PI 3-kinase/Akt and NF-kappaB activation in murine BV2 microglial cells. Neurosci Lett. 2006;396(1):1-6. doi:10.1016/j.neulet.2005.11.004
15. Martin L. Activation of the Adenosine A3 Receptor in RAW 264.7 Cells Inhibits Lipopolysaccharide-Stimulated Tumor Necrosis Factor- Release by Reducing Calcium-Dependent Activation of Nuclear Factor- B and Extracellular Signal-Regulated Kinase 1/2. J Pharmacol Exp Ther. 2005;316(1):71-78. doi:10.1124/jpet.105.091868
16. Shakibaei M, John T, Schulze-Tanzil G, Lehmann I, Mobasheri A. Suppression of NF-κB activation by curcumin leads to inhibition of expression of cyclo-oxygenase-2 and matrix metalloproteinase-9 in human articular chondrocytes: Implications for the treatment of osteoarthritis. Biochem Pharmacol. 2007;73(9):1434-1445. doi:10.1016/j.bcp.2007.01.005
17. De Mattei M, Varani K, Masieri FF, et al. Adenosine analogs and electromagnetic fields inhibit prostaglandin E2 release in bovine synovial fibroblasts. Osteoarthritis Cartilage. 2009;17(2):252-262. doi:10.1016/j.joca.2008.06.002
18. Vincenzi F, Targa M, Corciulo C, et al. Pulsed electromagnetic fields increased the anti-inflammatory effect of A_2A and A_3 adenosine receptors in human T/C-28a2 chondrocytes and hFOB 1.19 osteoblasts. PloS One. 2013;8(5):e65561. doi:10.1371/journal.pone.0065561
19. Ongaro A, Varani K, Masieri FF, et al. Electromagnetic fields (EMFs) and adenosine receptors modulate prostaglandin E 2 and cytokine release in human osteoarthritic synovial fibroblasts. J Cell Physiol. 2012;227(6):2461-2469. doi:10.1002/jcp.22981
20. Ongaro A, Pellati A, Setti S, et al. Electromagnetic fields counteract IL-1 β activity during chondrogenesis of bovine mesenchymal stem cells: EMFs counteract IL-1 β during chondrogenesis. J Tissue Eng Regen Med. 2015;9(12):E229-E238. doi:10.1002/term.1671
21. Parate D, Franco-Obregón A, Fröhlich J, et al. Enhancement of mesenchymal stem cell chondrogenesis with short-term low intensity pulsed electromagnetic fields. Sci Rep. 2017;7(1):9421. doi:10.1038/

s41598-017-09892-w
22. Wu L, Leijten JCH, Georgi N, Post JN, van Blitterswijk CA, Karperien M. Trophic Effects of Mesenchymal Stem Cells Increase Chondrocyte Proliferation and Matrix Formation. Tissue Eng Part A. 2011;17(9-10):1425-1436. doi:10.1089/ten.tea.2010.0517
23. Maumus M, Jorgensen C, Noël D. Mesenchymal stem cells in regenerative medicine applied to rheumatic diseases: Role of secretome and exosomes. Biochimie. 2013;95(12):2229-2234. doi:10.1016/j.biochi.2013.04.017
24. Parate D, Kadir ND, Celik C, et al. Pulsed electromagnetic fields potentiate the paracrine function of mesenchymal stem cells for cartilage regeneration. Stem Cell Res Ther. 2020;11(1):46. doi:10.1186/s13287-020-1566-5
25. Ciombor DM, Aaron RK, Wang S, Simon B. Modification of osteoarthritis by pulsed electromagnetic field--a morphological study. Osteoarthritis Cartilage. 2003;11(6):455-462.
26. Fini M, Giavaresi G, Torricelli P, et al. Pulsed electromagnetic fields reduce knee osteoarthritic lesion progression in the aged Dunkin Hartley guinea pig. J Orthop Res. 2005;23(4):899-908. doi:10.1016/j.orthres.2005.01.008
27. Fini M, Torricelli P, Giavaresi G, et al. Effect of pulsed electromagnetic field stimulation on knee cartilage, subchondral and epyphiseal trabecular bone of aged Dunkin Hartley guinea pigs. Biomed Pharmacother. 2008;62(10):709-715. doi:10.1016/j.biopha.2007.03.001
28. Benazzo F, Cadossi M, Cavani F, et al. Cartilage repair with osteochondral autografts in sheep: Effect of biophysical stimulation with pulsed electromagnetic fields. J Orthop Res. 2008;26(5):631-642. doi:10.1002/jor.20530
29. Veronesi F, Cadossi M, Giavaresi G, et al. Pulsed electromagnetic fields combined with a collagenous scaffold and bone marrow concentrate enhance osteochondral regeneration: an in vivo study. BMC Musculoskelet Disord. 2015;16(1):233. doi:10.1186/s12891-015-0683-2
30. Stefani RM, Barbosa S, Tan AR, et al. Pulsed electromagnetic fields promote repair of focal articular cartilage defects with engineered osteochondral constructs. Biotechnol Bioeng. 2020;117(5):1584-1596. doi:10.1002/bit.27287
31. Giannini S, Buda R, Cavallo M, et al. Cartilage repair evolution in post-traumatic osteochondral lesions of the talus: From open field autologous chondrocyte to bone-marrow-derived cells transplantation. Injury. 2010;41(11):1196-1203. doi:10.1016/j.injury.2010.09.028
32. Cadossi M, Buda RE, Ramponi L, Sambri A, Natali S, Giannini S. Bone Marrow–derived Cells and Biophysical Stimulation for Talar Osteochondral Lesions: A Randomized Controlled Study. Foot Ankle Int. 2014;35(10):981-987. doi:10.1177/1071100714539660
33. Collarile M, Sambri A, Lullini G, Cadossi M, Zorzi C. Biophysical stimulation improves clinical results of matrix-assisted

autologous chondrocyte implantation in the treatment of chondral lesions of the knee. Knee Surg Sports Traumatol Arthrosc. Published online June 17, 2017. doi:10.1007/s00167-017-4605-8

34. Reilingh ML, van Bergen CJA, Gerards RM, et al. Effects of Pulsed Electromagnetic Fields on Return to Sports After Arthroscopic Debridement and Microfracture of Osteochondral Talar Defects: A Randomized, Double-Blind, Placebo-Controlled, Multicenter Trial. Am J Sports Med. 2016;44(5):1292-1300. doi:10.1177/0363546515626544
35. Cadossi M, Sambri A, Sandro G, Massari L. Effects of Pulsed Electromagnetic Fields After Debridement and Microfracture of Osteochondral Talar Defects: Letter to the Editor. Am J Sports Med. 2016;44(11):NP60-NP61. doi:10.1177/0363546516676453
36. 36. Harris JD, Siston RA, Pan X, Flanigan DC. Autologous Chondrocyte Implantation: A Systematic Review. J Bone Jt Surg-Am Vol. 2010;92(12):2220-2233. doi:10.2106/JBJS.J.00049
37. 37. Correa D, Somoza RA, Lin P, et al. Sequential exposure to fibroblast growth factors (FGF) 2, 9 and 18 enhances hMSC chondrogenic differentiation. Osteoarthritis Cartilage. 2015;23(3):443-453. doi:10.1016/j.joca.2014.11.013
38. 38. Mithoefer K, McAdams T, Williams RJ, Kreuz PC, Mandelbaum BR. Clinical Efficacy of the Microfracture Technique for Articular Cartilage Repair in the Knee: An Evidence-Based Systematic Analysis. Am J Sports Med. 2009;37(10):2053-2063. doi:10.1177/0363546508328414
39. 39. Somoza RA, Welter JF, Correa D, Caplan AI. Chondrogenic Differentiation of Mesenchymal Stem Cells: Challenges and Unfulfilled Expectations. Tissue Eng Part B Rev. 2014;20(6):596-608. doi:10.1089/ten.teb.2013.0771

CHAPTER 3

TREATMENT OF OSTEONECROSIS OF THE FEMORAL HEAD

Dante Dallari, Nicolandrea Del Piccolo, Martina Rocchi

SC Orthopedic Reconstructive Surgery and Innovative Techniques
Musculoskeletal Tissue Bank

IRCCS - Rizzoli Orthopaedic Institute – Bologna

Introduction

Osteonecrosis (ON) of the femoral head is a condition characterized, from the pathological-anatomy point of view, by the collapse of the skeletal architecture and the cartilaginous surface following the necrosis of the bone tissue of the femoral epiphysis and, from the clinical point of view, by pain and joint functional limitation. Pathogenesis is often multifactorial. The therapeutic approach in advanced forms is hip arthroprosthesis. However, despite the progress achieved in recent decades in terms of reliability and duration, in the osteonecrosis it presents a lower survival rate and greater complications than the implanted prostheses for other etiologies. In addition, often involving young patients with high functional demands and long life expectancy, implanting a joint prosthesis often required the need for subsequent revision surgeries. For all these reasons, it is essential to set up a correct diagnostic process that allows early diagnosis and choose the most appropriate therapeutic approach in relation to the etiology and staging of osteonecrosis.

Epidemiology

Described for the first time by Munro in 1738, osteonecrosis is a progressively debilitating lesion that leads to a compromission of the hip joint [1], with a risk of collapse of the femoral head that, three years after onset, is described in 70-80% cases by Mont in a case-control study conducted on 664 asymptomatic osteonecrosis (follow-up range 0.2-20 years)[2]. In 1993 ARCO (Association Internationale de Recherche sur la Circulation Osseous) proposed the more general term osteonecrosis (ON) to define the disease characterized by the death of bone tissue, regardless of the causes and pathogenesis [3].

Osteonecrosis is a relatively common disease, whose incidence is around 10-20 thousand new cases per year in the USA [1], affects young adults, age between 20 and 50 years (average age 38 years) [4] and mainly affects the male sex (M:F = 7:3) (5). In the US, osteonecrosis represents the cause of 10% of the 500,000 interventions of reconstruction of the articular surface (6) and 10-18% of the 250,000 interventions of arthroprosthesis (THA) [7-8].

Pathogenesis

There are still many question marks about the pathogenesis of non-traumatic osteonecrosis. However, thanks to molecular genetics and the identification of an increasing number of pathologies that predispose the development of ON, the number of idiopathic forms is decreasing.

Theories on pathogenesis can be divided into:

- cell theories or direct cytotoxic damage;
- extraosseus theories;
- intraosseous theories.

An example of direct cytotoxic damage is mediated by radio-chemiotherapy, prolonged corticosteroid therapy, or chronic alcohol consumption. Extraosseus mechanisms can be arterial or venous. The correlation between the interruption of arterial flow and osteonecrosis is clear in the traumatic form, e.g., for medial fractures of the femoral neck. Less evident is, however, for non-traumatic forms. Intravascular occlusion of the arterial district is often documented, but it is not certain whether this is the cause or effect of the pathogenetic mechanism. Venous stasis is another aspect often observed, but even in this case, it is not yet clear whether it has a stimulating role or if it is the consequence of the pathology.

Finally, the intraosseous mechanism can also be intravascular or extravascular. Intravascular damage is due to the formation of an embolus in the microcirculation, both gaseous (as in dysbarism) and solid (present, for example, in coagulopathies such as sickle cell anemia). The extravascular mechanism is substantially linked to the increase in intracortical pressure caused by edema or a possible hemorrhage that involves a reduction in blood flow.

Diagnosis

The clinical symptoms, anamnesis, and instrumental evaluation are the primary tools to diagnose, identify the degree of necrosis, and choose, finally, the most suitable type of treatment [9]. A careful anamnesis must be carried out to frame the clinical and etiological situation of the patient. First of all, it is necessary to distinguish the traumatic forms (fractures, dislocations..) and osteonecrosis with indirect etiology; in this second case, it is necessary to investigate the intake of drugs (corticosteroids, antiretrovirals..), predisposing systemic pathologies, as mentioned above, pregnancies and volitional habits (smoking, alcohol abuse ..). Afterward, the doctor is required to evaluate the pain (location, intensity, irradiation..) and the consequent daily limitations, also exploiting specific scores (e.g., Harris Hip Score - HHS). The patient's clinical picture is then essential to guide the therapeutic process. After observing the patient's walking and the possible asymmetry, the doctor must analyze passive and active motility: intra-rotation is often limited. In the most advanced stages, the remaining movements are also affected. For an accurate diagnosis, imaging is also crucial. The radiographic study is the first examination to be carried out and is performed in AP and LL projections. The RX images that are obtained often allow to evaluate well the extent of necrosis and the severity of the clinical picture. Magnetic resonance imaging is considered the most accurate investigation method to quantify the osteonecrotic area at an early stage and to identify the topographic site of the lesion, with a sensitivity ranging between 88 and 100% thanks to the characteristics of multiplanar and multiparametric. MRI also has the advantage of discriminating the bone component from the cartilaginous one, highlighting a possible chondropathy [10-11-12] (fig.1). MRI is the first choice for post-diagnosis and post-treatment monitoring and has an important role in screening subjects exposed to high risk. This technique has shown effectiveness in predicting the probability of collapse: Nishii, in a study, has shown that the

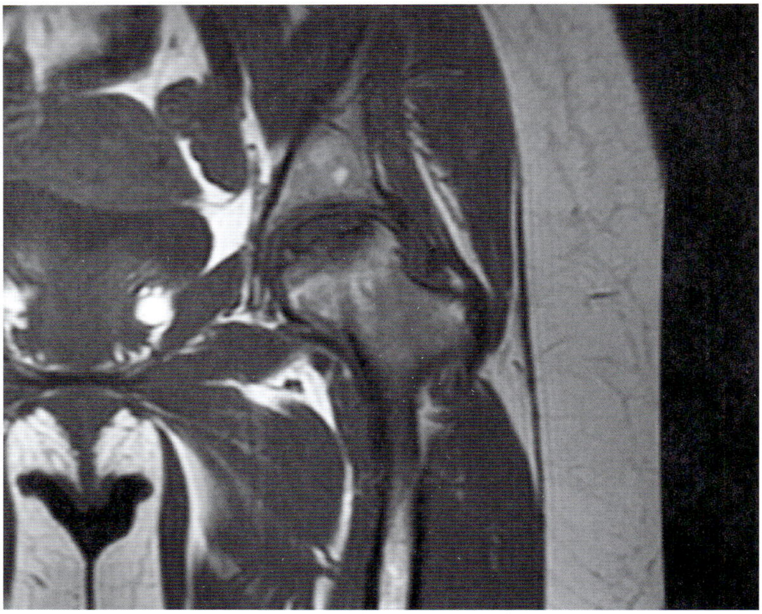

Figure 1 MRI showing signal hyperintensity in the osteonecrotic area and initial sphericity alteration of the epiphysis

risk is higher if more than 30% of the epiphysis is involved and the lesion is located in the anterosuperior region. Bone scintigraphy with Tc99 methylene diphosphonate has been used for years in the early diagnosis of osteonecrosis; however, due to its low specificity, it has been entirely replaced by the use of MRI [4].

Finally, CT can be used for a detailed evaluation of the affected area and joint microfractures in view of surgical treatment [13] but has a secondary role in the diagnosis in the early phase.

Classification

One of the fundamental obstacles to the study, diagnosis, and treatment of osteonecrosis is the lack of a universally shared classification system.

In the evaluation of a system for classifying ONs, several key points must

be taken into account:
MRI is a highly specific diagnostic method with a sensitivity ranging from 80% to 100%. The symptomatology is not an indicator of severity because it is variable and subjective; therefore, it is not part of a classification system. The size of necrosis: it is an important prognostic factor. However, the best method of measurement remains to be defined. The presence of epiphyseal collapse at the time of diagnosis: is considered the primary negative prognostic indicator, denoting the irreversibility of the pathology. The involvement of the acetabular is an indicator of the severity of the pathology. The best evaluation method has not yet been clarified. The lesion localization is less important than the size [13-14-15].
The first classification dates back in the 60s, before the advent of MRI, and was created by Arlet-Ficat: it was based on radiographic evaluation, originally consisting of three stages, in 1980 a fourth stage was introduced to indicate joint involvement and, finally, in 1985, the zero stage was added, defined as pre-clinical and pre-radiographic, with reduced uptake at scintigraphy.
The classification developed most recently to understand these elements is the Arco (Association Research Circulation Osseous) classification, drawn in 1991, to create the most complete and reproducible classification system, using radiographic images, MRI, bone scintigraphy, and histological findings. The progression of osteonecrosis is divided into 5 stages, including the zero stage, which is pre-radiographic (fig.2).

Conservative treatment

The purpose of the treatment of osteonecrosis is to prevent the disease's progression and achieve the regression of the symptomatology [16]. There are numerous proposed treatments, the choice of the most adequate one depends on the stage, extent, localization, and etiology of necrosis. The results, guaranteed by conservative treatments, are still poorly defined; however, the importance of early diagnosis and precise staging of the lesion is

Stage	Characteristics	Location
0	Bone biopsy compatible with avascular necrosis; other normal tests	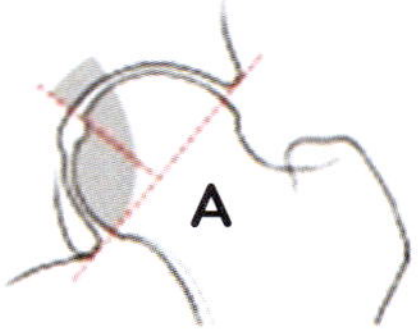
I	Bone scintigraphy and positive MRI; the lesions are further classified into medial, central or lateral depending on the location in the femoral head	Medial 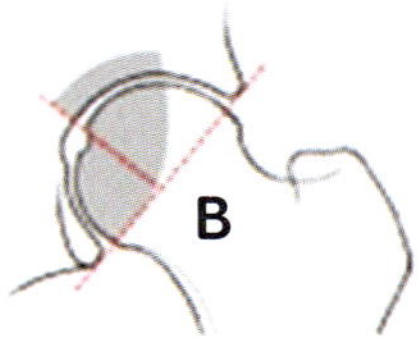
I-A	Involvement of the femoral head <15%*	
I-B	Involvement of the femoral head 15-30%*	
I-C	Involvement of the femoral head >30%*	
II	II Radiographic anomalies (mottled schlerotic femoral head, osteosclerosis, cysts and osteopenia); no sign of femoral head collapse at X-rays or CT; bone scintigraphy and positive MRI; any acetabular alteration; lesions divided into medial, central and lateral	Central 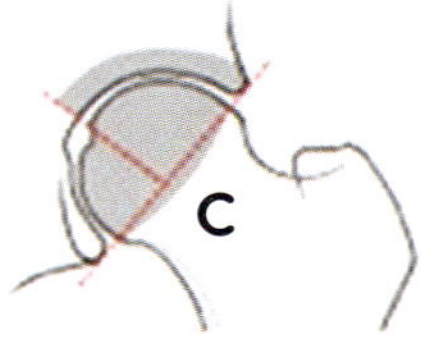
II-A	Involvement of the femoral head <15%*	
II-B	Involvement of the femoral head 15-30%*	
II-C	Involvement of the femoral head >30%*	Lateral **Involvement**
III	Crescent shape: the lesions are further classified into medial, central or lateral depending on the location in the femoral head	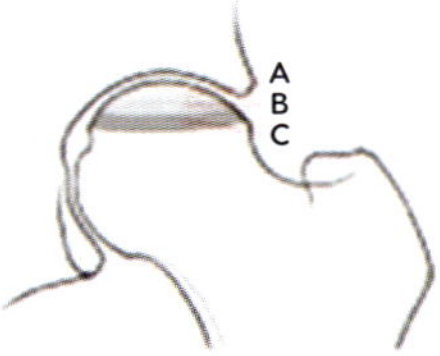
III-A	Crescent shape <15% or depression of the femoral head <2 mm**	
III-B	Crescent shape 15-30% % or depression of the femoral head 2-4 mm**	**A:** < 15% < 2 mm
III-C	Crescent shape 30% or depression of the femoral head >4mm**	**B:** 15-30%
IV	Joint surface of flattened appearance and reduced joint space to the x-ray; acetabular changes with evidence of osteosclerosis; marginal cysts and osteophytes	**C:** >30% >4 mm

* MRI
** X-rays in front-rear and side projection (adapted from Mont.1995)

Figure 2 ARCO classification

crucial to intervene before the collapse of the epiphysis, a sign of irreversible impairment of the coxo-femoral joint. In the most advanced forms, the only therapeutic option of symptoms and disability is the prosthetic replacement of the hip.

The suspension of the load obtained thanks to antibrachial sticks has been proposed in early injuries. In a meta-analysis carried out on 819 patients, Mont shows, however, that in 80% of patients, in a 34 months of follow-up, there is no significant difference between those who observed a period of discharge, complete or partial, compared to patients who had no limitations [2]. Hyperbaric oxygen therapy and the use of vasodilated prostacyclin analogs (Iloprost) have been shown to affect bone marrow bone tissue edema in cases of early-stage necrosis. However, only studies with limited, uncontrolled samples are available. The rationale for using bisphosphonates in the treatment of osteonecrosis is to slow down the resorption of necrotic bone, inhibit osteoclasts, and allow the formation of new bone tissue before the collapse of the epiphysis occurs. Hernigou, in a study on the natural history of untreated osteonecrosis, showed that this is evolving in 70% of cases towards the collapse of normal anatomy after an average of 3.5 years in stage I and 2.9 in stage II; this rate is favorably altered by the use of bisphosphonates, in particular by Alendronate [17]. Similar results have been highlighted by several studies [18]. However, in the literature, there are discordant articles on the effectiveness of the therapy.

In stage I-II osteonecrosis, associated with thrombophilic and hypofibrinolysis states, a possibility of bloodless treatment is offered by the use of Enoxaparin [19]. However, in this case, side effects have also been limiting its application, especially for numerous cases of thrombocytopenias induced by heparin and by the possible osteoporosis induced by the drug [20].

Pulsed electromagnetic fields (EMPs) have proved useful, as a biophysical stimulus, in bone tissue repair phenomena, and a chondroprotective effect has also recently been demonstrated. (21).

However, the evidence in favor is still rather limited, and further studies are needed to clarify the role of PEMFs therapy in preventing disease progression [22]. Extracorporeal shock waves are a physical treatment method that has been shown to help promote bone repair and reduce painful symptoms in some insertional tendinopathies. In a randomized clinical trial in Stage I-II and 38 III Arco patients, Wang highlights the superiority of clinical and radiographic outcomes in shock wave patients compared to those undergoing decompression and non-vascularized grafts following 24 months of follow-up [23]. However, the average follow-up of the study (24 months) is insufficient to draw certain conclusions over the medium to long term [24]. The mechanism by which such a method would act is not entirely clear.

Surgical treatment

Core Decompression (CD) or outbreak decompression is the surgical procedure historically most used to treat the early stages of osteonecrosis, introduced by Ficat and Arlet in the 60s. Observing increased intramedullary pressures and delayed sinusoidal venous drainage in the proximal femur, Ficat and Arlet developed the hypothesis that vascular stasis and prolonged ischemia were involved in the pathogenesis of avascular necrosis. Core Decompression aims to decompress the femoral head and, consequently, reduce intraosseous pressure to restore normal vascular flow. This condition should promote osteogenesis in the area of the lesion. Despite being one of the most proven surgical techniques, there is still no real consensus in the literature about it, nor clarity on indications and long-term results; it remains, therefore, controversial whether this procedure really affects the natural evolution of the disease.

A further therapeutic possibility is represented by using non-vascularized bone grafts through impaction grafting or bone substitutes to be associated with decompression. The rationale of the two techniques is to offer mechanical support to the subchondral bone stimulating osteogenesis and neoangiogenesis. The bone grafts used are made up of spongy or corticospongious bone. They can be homologous or autologous, obtained from the tibia, the iliac crest, or the trochanteric region if you use a single incision. Recent acquisitions in the field of the pathophysiology of osteonecrosis suggest that a reduction in the pool of mesenchymal cells in the proximal region of the femur leads to a decrease in osteoblasts and a consequent deficit in the phenomena of remodeling and regeneration of the bone; it has been, for this reason, hypothesized that the best results, obtained with autologous tibial grafts compared to those coming from the trochanter, are to be related to the different site of the collection, in addition to the greater amount of grafting that the tibial metaphysis can provide [25]. The results of decompression associated with bone grafts are satisfactory in stage II lesions, according to Ficat [26]; in the phases following the collapse of the anatomy of the epiphysis, these methods cannot return sphericity to the head and consequently are not indicated in the ON stage III-IV. The evolution of these decompression techniques and non-vascularized grafts consists of increasing the regenerative potential using autologous growth factors or concentrated autologous stromal cells, without substantially modifying the surgical technique. Lieberman et al. describe positive results thanks to treatment with purified human BMPs (bone morphogenetic proteins): 4 years after surgery, 82% (14/18) of patients did not undergo prosthetic replacement [27]. In his prospective study, Gangji points out a significant reduction in pain and local symptoms in patients treated with decompression and autologous stromal cells, compared to the control group treated with decompression alone, and notes the effectiveness of the method in delaying the evolution towards stage III to a follow-up of 2 years. Ganjii, in particular, highlights the possible tendency to the reversibility of the lesion: the percentage of volume of necrotic tissue was reduced by 35% in the stromal cell group, while it increased, on average, by 23% in the control group.

In addition to the increased regenerative potential offered by stromal cells, one possible explanation would lie in the secretion of angiogenic cytokines by the cells themselves [28]. In reality, the use of stromal cells does not significantly delay the total prosthesis compared to core decompression alone. However, it gives a considerable symptomatic relief and a more evident success from the radiological and clinical point of view, evaluated through HHS [29].

Vascularized bone grafts are based on an autologous bone fragment with a muscular peduncle. Judet was the first to introduce its use in femoral neck fractures [30]. Subsequently, Meyers and Palazzi proposed a similar procedure for the treatment of stage I-II osteonecrosis according to Ficat, which involves the use of spongy bone of the iliac crest positioned in a bony trench, dug into the neck, up to the subchondral bone, and covered by a muscular peduncle, obtained from the square of the femur. Meyers describes satisfactory results both in terms of pain resolution and stopping the progression of the disease. However, such a procedure is not able to offer sufficient mechanical support to the subchondral bone. Recently, an increasing number of studies report promising results thanks to the use of autologous vascularized fibula; the rationale for the intervention is based on the following principles:

- the decompression effect on the femoral head;
- the removal of necrotic tissue;
- the mechanical supporting effect of the subchondral bone;
- the biological stimulus to revascularization and neoangiogenesis in the infarcted region [31].

Malizos describes good results in 100% of cases with osteonecrosis stage II-III according to Steinberg. In a study by Urbaniak, the results were satisfactory, i.e., the need to perform an arthroprosthesis following a minimum follow-up of 5 years did not arise, in 89% of patients in Stage II, in 77% in stage III, in 57% in stage IV and 68% in stage V. Urbaniak highlights the importance of possible joint degeneration at the time of surgery: in the group of patients, who radiologically manifest the collapse of the subchondral bone, the success rate is equal to 85%, but drops to 73% if the narrowing of the articular rhyme is concomitant. Other fundamental factors for the prognosis are the patient's medical history, particularly volitional habits, such as alcohol and smoking and vascular pathologies, which must be investigated compulsorily before the procedure [32]. Despite the encouraging results, the complexity of the intervention, the extended surgical times, and the morbidity at the donor site make this procedure scarcely popular. The indication, for young and symptomatic patients, without collapse of the subchondral bone, maybe controversial because, in these subjects, the results of more straightforward procedures are equally encouraging. Currently, there are no prospective, randomized and controlled studies in the literature that compare the technique of vascularized grafts with other less investigative interventions [33-34].

An alternative to the bone grafts associated with the decompression of the femoral head is represented by the use of artificial devices that perform a mechanical support action of the subchondral bone. These systems provide for the placement of cylindrical structures manufactured with biomaterials, which can be screwed into the neck and proximal epiphysis of the femur to support the necrotic area after careful curettage. One of the most common biomaterials is represented by tantalum, characterized by a trabecular structure that integrates well into the host bone and endowed with a modulus of elasticity similar to the skeletal one, such as to avoid stress-shielding phenomena. The objectives to be achieved through this conservative surgical technique consist in restoring the anatomy, allowing the revascularization of the proximal femoral epiphysis, and avoiding or postponing a more invasive intervention. In the literature, no randomized clinical trials are analyzing the long-term results of these methods [35].

The rationale for femoral osteotomy interventions in the treatment of osteonecrosis is to reduce the load stress on the necrotic area to decrease the progression of the disease and, possibly, induce the healing of the lesion. There are two main techniques: angular osteotomy and rotational osteotomy. In 1969 Schneider proposed an intertrochanteric flexural osteotomy aimed at rotating the intact back of the femoral head towards the part of the acetabulum responsible for loading; this technique has become very popular due to its effectiveness, which is ensured if the osteotomy is carefully programmed and carried out in highly selected patients. Scher and Jakim [36] report the results of valgus-flexion osteotomies carried out in 45 patients suffering from osteonecrosis stage III Arco, under the age of 45 years, in the absence of systemic diseases: the percentage of joint survival, at 5 years, was equal to 87%. Overall, from the analysis of the cases published in the literature on the techniques of femoral osteotomy in the treatment of osteonecrosis, it is clear that the results are difficult to compare due to the different indications to this intervention and often not entirely predictable. In addition, there are no comparative trials between this technique, CD, and bone grafts resulting in insufficient data to draw exhaustive conclusions on the indications and prognosis of treatment. Numerous reviews, however, show that the outcome of the intervention depends on the pathogenesis of the disease, the stage and extent of the osteonecrosis, the general clinical picture, and the degree of preoperative motility. These methods are more reliable in necrosis, not secondary to metabolic pathologies or the intake of GC or chemotherapeutic agents, in stages IIIII according to Ficat, when the preoperative arc of movement is normal or slightly reduced [5].

The implantation of a joint prosthesis aims to replace the articular surface with the least possible bone sacrifice. Techniques include lining prosthesis or total arthroprosthesis. Prosthetic coating surgery is a much-discussed therapeutic option for survival and release of ions. Several studies underline the non-correlation between the survival of the prosthesis and extension of the pre-application osteonecrosis and demonstrate excellent results in the long term. Total arthroprosthesis surgery offers an immediate solution to pain and a rapid functional recovery. The literature seems to partly penalize the total arthroprostheses carried out in patients suffering from osteonecrosis in long-term follow-ups, compared to those implanted for primary or secondary osteoarthritis, due to the younger age of the patient and, therefore, the longer survival and functionality required [37-38-39]. Overall, long-term outcomes tend to deteriorate in patients under 50, particularly under 30. Better results were highlighted with new cementation techniques or in non-cemented prostheses, thanks to the use of new materials made of high molecular weight polyethylene and ceramic couplings on ceramics. Although the cases are limited, the literature suggests using increased implants and innovative materials in young patients and, in any case, if the bone is of good quality [40].

In the experience of the Rizzoli Orthopaedic Institute, the ceramic-ceramic coupling, especially in young patients, has proven to be reliable and has made it possible to minimize the effects of wear and tear on materials. Some subgroups of patients with secondary osteonecrosis (alcoholics, obese patients, or undergoing chronic corticosteroid therapy) are burdened with an increased risk of failure due to aseptic or septic mobilization; in particular, a correlation was found between severe alcoholism and periprosthetic femoral fractures [41-42]. However, the development of implantation techniques and materials have led in the last decade to results in survival and fewer very encouraging complications, as shown by several studies: - Chang et al. demonstrate an average life of total prosthetic implants, at 10.2 years of follow-up, in patients undergoing renal transplantation in the norm [43]. - a second positive example is proposed by the Issa group that compares, in a case-control study, patients suffering from sickle cell anemia and osteonecrosis treated with protein replacement: at 7 years, there were no higher rates, compared to subjects suffering from only osteonecrosis, of septic and non-septic complications (95% against 97%).

Personal case series

One of the several researches of the SC of Orthopedic Reconstructive Surgery and Innovative Techniques (CORTI, in the past Orthopedic and Traumatological Clinic I) of the Rizzoli Orthopedic Institute aims at the study of the pathophysiology of osteonecrosis and the treatment of this pathology through the use of regenerative medicine techniques. The experience began in 2002, with studies conducted on laboratory animals to evaluate the efficacy of autologous platelet gel (PRP) and concentrated autologous stromal cells (BMSCs). The results of this trial were encouraging because both PRP and BMSCs have been shown to play an important role in promoting bone regeneration [44]. This analysis continued with a randomized, double-blind study in patients undergoing tibial osteotomy. The results obtained showed better osseointegration of the grafts adjuvant with PRP and/or BMSC, also confirmed by statistical tests [45-46]. Thanks to the results achieved, autologous adjuvants have begun to be used in clinical practice for the treatment of pseudo-arthrosis of long bones, in hip prosthetic reimplants with large losses of bone substance, and in the osteonecrosis of the femoral head. Concerning the latter pathology, the attention was initially focused on stage II according to the Arco classification, that is, on the early pictures in which the cartilage has not been involved yet and, inspired by the experience of Hernigou and Gangji, Core Decompression and bone graft techniques were used with grafts of freeze-dried homologous bone added with PRP and BMSC. Subsequently, it was decided to extend the treatment indications to pictures with more advanced joint impairment.

Core decompression: surgical technique

- I° step: the patient is positioned in supine decubitus with the hip 5 to 10° intra-rotated, in order to place the femoral neck parallel to the floor. Once the operating field is set up, a bone marrow blood sample is taken from the homolateral anterior iliac crest and the concentration of autologous stromal cells is obtained (BMSC).

- II° step: after evaluating the level of trans-trochanteric access with a Kirschner thread under amplioscopic control, a skin incision of about 3 cm is made. A dedicated instrument is used to perform a percutaneous perforation up to about 11 mm in diameter on the cervical axis directed to the area of cephalic necrosis and prolonged up to the subchondral bone portion under amplioscopic control. In the case of large necrotic lesions, we proceed with the same technique in the adjacent areas, possibly with perforators of smaller diameter, until the pathological area is cleared (fig. 3). The samples, thus obtained, are sent to the laboratory for histological analysis. At the same time, the

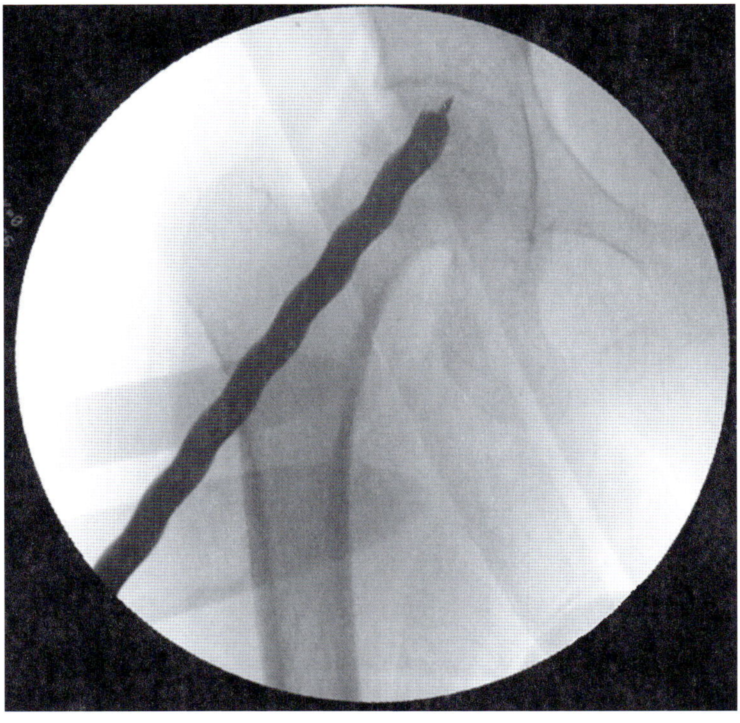

Figure 3 Core Decompression

assistant proceeds to the assembly of the BMSC previously obtained with lyophilized homologous bone chips and autologous platelet gel (PRP) produced the previous day at the transfusion service.

- III° step : therefore, this preparation is used to seal ,with a beater, the hole left by the removal of the necrosis area and the decompression. The surgical access is sutured, and the placement of surgical drains is usually not necessary.

The postoperative program may vary depending on the patient's age, weight, and collaboration. Typically, the partial load is not indicated earlier than 45 days; the total load is allowed at 3 months.

Core Decompression results

Following this technique, between 2005 and 2018, we treated 112 necrosis of the femoral head in 103 patients. The mean age of the treated patient group was 38.3 years (16-62), and the prevalence of male patients over female patients was 78 and 34 cases. At the moment of surgery, 50% of the cases treated had already advanced necrosis of Arco 3 stage, 40.8% were in Arco 2 while few cases were Arco 1 (1.92%) and Arco 4 (7.69%).

The results at an average follow-up of 49.4 months (range 13-116) showed a strong correlation between the stage of necrosis and the treatment failure, with the need for prosthetic replacement. This was necessary for 57% of Arco 3 patients and only 23% of Arco 2 patients. The clinical evaluation of the successes has also shown a high percentage of good/excellent results in patients who have maintained good values of a joint function over time.

Osteochondral repair

The bad results obtained in Arco 3 cases have led us to develop a non-prosthetic surgical treatment dedicated to managing joint involvement of the pathology. Drawing inspiration from knee surgery, engineered autologous cartilage implantation techniques and bioceramic cylinders (TruFit) have been applied to hip surgery. The TruFit system is an implant consisting of a cylindrical plug of different sizes inserted inside the osteochondral defect, acting as a scaffolding that protects the integrity of the surrounding tissues, preventing further collapse and progression of the defect. The device also represents a resorbable substrate, morphologically and physically suitable to support cell migration and growth to repair osteochondral defects.

An original surgical technique was used, devised by Ganz [47], to access the joint while preserving the vascularization of the proximal femoral epiphysis and, therefore, reducing the ischemic complications that would aggravate the osteonecrosis. As well demonstrated, the artery of the round ligament participates to an extremely low extent in the vascularization of the femoral head. At the same time, from studies carried out by the Swiss School, the vascular contribution is determined mainly by the medial femoral circumflex. The goal is, therefore, the respect of this artery.

Osteochondral repair surgical technique

- I° step: once the operating field is set up, a bone marrow blood sample is taken from the homolateral anterior iliac crest and autologous stromal cells (BMSC) concentration is obtained.
- II° step: a lateral access is obtained with the Kocher-Langenbeck type section of the fascia lata and a couple of centimeters from the distal trochanteric insertion of the middle gluteus. We then proceed with the proximal intermuscular dissection of the same muscle and with the isolation of the tendon of the small gluteus, which is detached about 0.5 cm from its trochanteric insertion. Once the joint capsule is exposed, the incision must be made in order to dislocate the epiphysis. Hip dislocation

is a rare occurrence in orthopedic surgery due to the high risk of the maneuver to interrupt the vascularization of the femoral head; despite this, the broad vision that is offered to us, through this access, allows us not only to explore the bone and cartilage anatomy of the epiphysis, but, also, to intervene in a precise and direct way in pathologies such as rheumatoid synovitis, chondromatosis and, of course, ON. In our experience, we used a modification of the technique described by Ganz with an S-incision of the joint capsule to protect the vascularization of the femoral head.

- III° step: dislocated the epiphysis, the area of necrosis is highlighted, treated until the vital spongy bone is exposed. An assistant proceeds, in the meantime, to the assembly of the adjuvants and homologous and synthetic grafts used: the lyophilized bone chips and the selected biomaterials are immersed in the concentrated bone marrow cells for a minimum time of 30'.
- IV step: with a special instrument, we then proceed to dig a housing-hole for the biomaterials in the femoral epiphysis (fig. 4). After applying the biomaterials, the homologous bone chips are used to fill the spaces returning homogeneous sphericity of the femoral epiphysis. The area is finally coated with a chondroinductive membrane soaked in BMSC, stabilized with resorbable sutures. Subsequently, the epiphysis is reduced, and the capsule and gluteal musculature are carefully sutured.

Postoperative rehabilitation included a program of progressive mobilization exercises aimed at recovering joint ROM and walking with a load protected with antibrachial sticks for the first 3 months after surgery.

Osteochondral repair results

We also performed this procedure 26 times (24 patients) with an average age of 32 years (18-44). The sample mainly includes male patients (19 males, 5 females). The etiology of necrosis in 10

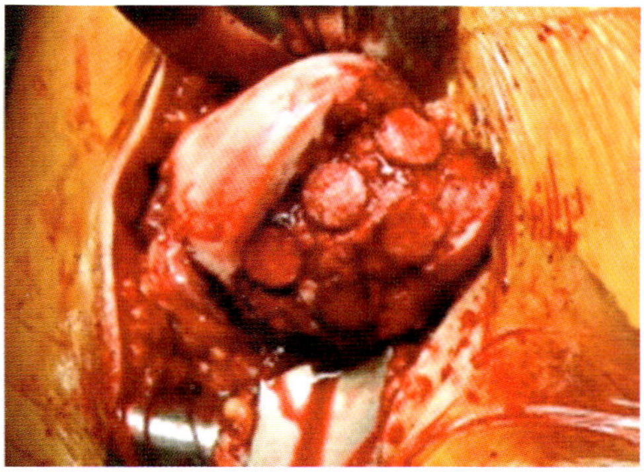

Figure 4 Implantation of biomaterials in osteochondral repair

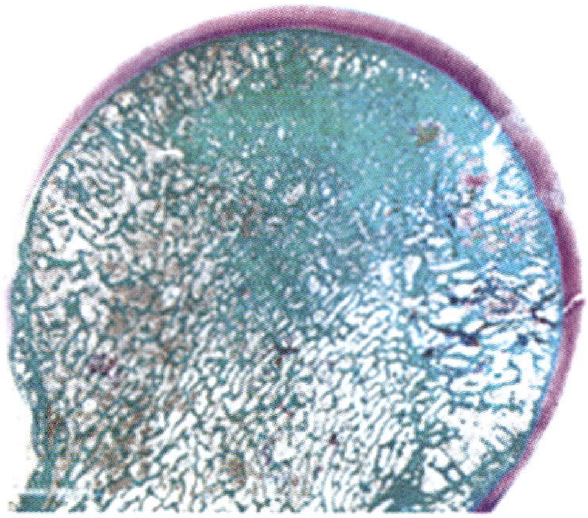

Figure 5 Histological result 5 years after osteochondral repair. Overview of the histological section of the femoral head. Presence of cartilage tissue (purple) along the entire articular surface. Presence of thickening areas bone not distinguishable from the underlying bone. It is possible to detect the presence of rare residues of material

post-traumatic cases (6 femoral neck fractures and 4 traumatic luxations). Of the non-post-traumatic cases, the causative agent was identified in steroid therapy (4 cases), while in the remaining 12 cases, necrosis was idiopathic.

From a clinical point of view, the procedure failed to guarantee an improvement in symptomatology in 15 of the cases. It was necessary to perform a subsequent hip prosthesis surgery at an average distance from the intervention of 25.7 months (7-78). The remaining patients had an initial improvement in clinic function test scores (mean HHS from 48.37 to 82.61) which was maintained until a mean follow-up of 82.3 months (52-125). The histological analysis of the failed cases has shown excellent osseointegration of the biological system (fig. 5). However, morphological studies, obtained through micro-CT and 3D reconstructions, have highlighted a severe deficit of the morphology of the femoral epiphysis (fig. 6), which has predisposed the joint to a rapid arthritic degeneration, probable cause of the need for prosthetic replacement.

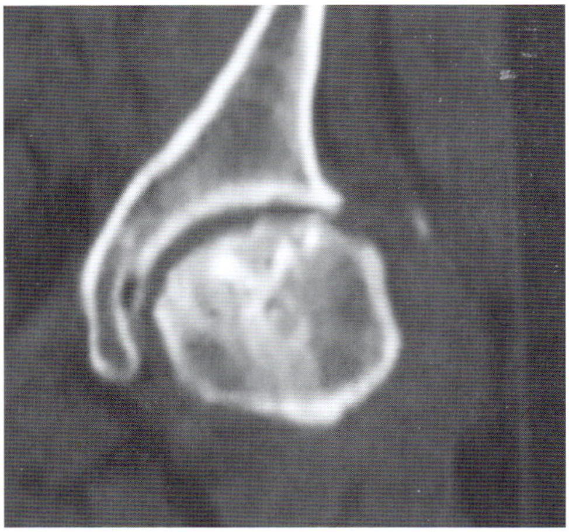

Figure 6 Result at 5 years of follow-up after osteochondral reconstruction (CT image)

Conclusions

Osteonecrosis of the femoral head is a frequent pathology that involves considerable social costs, due to the need to perform prosthesis in young patients, with a consequent reduction in their working capacity, the impossibility of practicing certain types of activities, and a high probability that, over the years, several prosthetic revisions will be necessary.

Core Decompression of the necrotic area associated with the implantation of homologous grafts and biological adjuvants (PRP and BMSC) is a procedure characterized by low morbidity that allows to avoid or postpone the need for a hip prosthetic replacement intervention in a high percentage of patients. The indication of choice is in the forms of necrosis of the femoral head that do not present depressions of the articular surface in Arco 2 degrees or Arco 3 degrees with involvement of up to one-third of the articular surface.

The most advanced cases treated with intra-articular reconstructive procedures have given inconstant results due to the difficulty in reconstructing the morphology of the articular epiphysis even if the use of the association of biomaterials and bone grafts with biological adjuvants have shown a good potentiality in the reconstruction of subchondral bone tissue and cartilage tissue.

The use of new custom-shaped scaffolds could represent an exciting prospect in this clinical application.

References

1. Mont MA, Hungerford DS: Non traumatic avascular necrosis of the femorale head. J Bon Joint Am 1995;77: 459-474.
2. Mont MA, Zywiel MG, Marker DR, et al. The natural history of untreated asymp-

tomatic osteonecrosis of the femoral head: a systematic literature review. The Journal of bone and joint surgery American volume 2010;92:2165–70.

3. Malizos KN, Karantanas AH, Varitimidis SE, et al : Osteonecrosis of the femoral head: etiology, imaging and treatment. Eur J Radiol 2007; 63:16-28.
4. Carlos J. Lavernia, MD, Rafael J. Sierra, and Francisco R. Grieco, MD: Osteonecrosis of the femoral Head. J Am Acad Orthop Surg 1999;7: 250-261.
5. Yerudith Assouline-Dayan, Christopher Chang, Adam Greenspan, Yehuda Shoenfeld, and M. Eric Gerhwin: Pathogenesis and Natural History of Osteonecrosis. Semin Arthritis Rheum 2002;32:94-124.
6. MankinHJ: Nontraumatic necrosis of bone (osteonecrosis). N. Engl J Med 1992; 326: 1473-9.
7. Paul E. Beaulé, MD, FRCSC, and Harlan C. Amstutz, MD: Management of Ficat Stage III and IV Osteonecrosis of the Hip. J Am Acad Orthop Surg 2004; 12:96-105.
8. Dabov G, Perez EA. Osteonecrosis. In: ST channel, editor. Campbell's operative orthopaedics. 10th ed. Philadelphia USA: Mosby; 2002. p.946-57.
9. Steinberg ME, Bands RE, Parry S, et al: Does lesion size affect the out come in avascular necrosis? Clin Orthop 1999; 262-271.
10. Saini A, Saifuddin A: MRI of osteonecrosis. 2004; 59:1079-1093
11. Nakamuta T, Matsumoto T, Nishino M, et al: Early Magnetic resonance imaging and histologic findings in a model of femoral head necrosis. Clin Orthop 1997; 334:68-72.
12. Sakamoto M, Shimizu K, Akita T, et al: Osteonecrosis of the femoral head: A prospective study with MRI. J Bone Joint Surg Br 1997;79:213-219
13. Steinberg ME, Hayken GD, Steinberg DR: A quantitative system for staging avascular necrosis. J Bone Joint Surg Br. 1995;77:34-41.
14. Michael A, Mont, German A, et al: Systematic Analysis of Classification System for Osteonecrosis of the Femoral Head. J Bone Joint Surg Am 2006;88:16-26.
15. 15. Gardeniers JWM. A new International classification of osteonecrosis of the ARCO committee on terminology and classification. ARCO News Letter 1992;4:41-6.
16. Ficat RP, Arlet J: Ischemia and Necrosis of bone. Baltimore. Williams and Wilkins, 1980, pp 29-52.
17. Hernigou P, Poignard A, Nogier A, et al. Fate of very small asymptomatic stage-I osteonecrotic lesions of the hip. The Journal of bone and joint surgery American volume 2004;86-A:2589–93.
18. Lai KA, Shen WJ, Yang CY, et al. The use of alendr- onate to prevent early collapse of the femoral head in patients with nontraumatic osteonecrosis. A randomized clinical study. The Journal of bone and joint surgery American volume 2005;87:2155–9.
19. Glueck CJ, Freiberg RA, Sieve L, et al. Enoxaparin prevents progression of stages I and II osteonecro- sis of the hip.

Clinical orthopaedics and related research 2005;164–7.
20. Massari, Fini, Cadossi, et al: Biophysical stimulation with pulsed electromagnetic fields in osteonecrosis of the femoral head. J Bone Joint Surg 2006;3:48-55
21. Steinberg ME, Brighton CT, Corces A, et al: Osteonecrosis of the femoral head results of core decompression bone grafting with and without electrical stimulation. Clin Orthop Relates Res. 1989;249:199-208.
22. Massari L, Fini M, Cadossi R, et al. Biophysical stimulation with pulsed electromagnetic fields in osteonecrosis of the femoral head. The Journal of bone and joint surgery American volume 2006; 88(Suppl 3):56–60.
23. Wang CJ, Huang CC, Wang JW, et al. Long-term results of extracorporeal shockwave therapy and core decompression in osteonecrosis of the femoral head with eight- to nine-year follow-up. Biomedical journal 2012;35:481–5.
24. Wang Ching-Jen, Wnag Feng-Sheng, Huang Chung- Cheng, et al: Treatment of Osteonecrosis of the femoral head: Comparison of Extracorporeal Shock Waves with Core Decompression and Bone Grafting. J Bone Joint Surg Am 2005;87:2380-2387.
25. Keizer SB, Kock NB, Dijkstra, et al: Treatment of avascular necrosis of the hip by non vascularised cortical graft. J Bone Joint Surg Br 2006;88:460-6.
26. Castro FP, Jr., Barrack RL: Core decompression and conservative treatment for avascular necrosis of the femoral head: a meta-analysis. Am J Orthop 2000;29:187-194.
27. Lieberman JR, Conduah A, Urist MR. Treatment of osteonecrosis of the femoral head with core decompression and human bone morphogenetic protein. Clinical orthopaedics and related research 2004;139–45.
28. Gangji Valerie and Hauzeur Jean Philippe: Treatment of osteonecrosis of the Femoral Head with implantation of autologous Marrow Cells. J Bone Joint Surg Am 2005;87:106-112.
29. Gangji V, De Maertelaer V, Hauzeur JP. Autologous bone marrow cell implantation in the treatment of non-traumatic osteonecrosis of the femoral head: Five year follow-up of a prospective controlled study. Bone 2011;49:1005–9.
30. Judet H, Gilbert A: Long term results of free vascularised fibular grafting for femoral head necrosis. Clin Orthop Relat Res 2001;386:114-9.
31. Meyers MH: The treatment of osteonecrosis of the hip with fresh osteochondral allograft and with the muscle pedicle graft technique. Clin Orthop 1978; 130:202-9.
32. Urbaniak JR, Coogan PG, Gunneson EB, et al. Treatment of osteonecrosis of the femoral head with free vascularized fibular grafting. A long-term follow-up study of one hundred and three hips. The Journal of bone and joint surgery American volume 1995;77:681–94.
33. Urbaniak JR. Aseptic necrosis of the femoral head treated by vascularised fibular graft. Microsurgery for major limb

reconstruction. St. Louis: CV Mosby, 1987:178-84.

34. Aldridge JM 3rd, Berend KR, Gunneson EE, et al: Free vascularised fibular grafting for the treatment of postcollapse osteonecrosis of the femoral head. J Bone Joint Surg Am 2004;86-A:87-101.
35. Nadeau M, Seguin C, Theodoropoulus JS: Short Term Clinical outcome of a porous tantalum implant for the treatment of advanced osteonecrosis of the femoral head. Mc Gill J Med 2007;10:4-10.
36. Briggs WA, Hampers CL, Merril Jp, et al: Aseptic necrosis in the femur after transplantation. Ann Surg 1972; 175: 282-289.
37. Issa K, Naziri Q, Rasquinha VJ, et al. Outcomes of Primary Total Hip Arthroplasty in Systemic Lupus Erythematosus With a Proximally-Coated Cement- less Stem. The Journal of arthroplasty 2013
38. Issa K, Johnson AJ, Naziri Q, et al. Hip Osteonec- rosis: Does Prior Hip Surgery Alter Outcomes Compared to an Initial Primary Total Hip Arthro- plasty? The Journal of arthroplasty 2013.
39. Issa K, Naziri Q, Maheshwari AV, et al. Excellent Results and Minimal Complications of Total Hip Arthroplasty in Sickle Cell Hemoglobinopathy at Mid-Term Follow-Up Using Cementless Prosthetic Components. The Journal of arthroplasty 2013.
40. Mont MA, Ragland PS, Etienne G. Core decom pression of the femoral head for osteonecrosis using percutaneous multiple small-diameter drilling. Clinical orthopaedics and related research 2004; 131–8.
41. Adili A, Trousdale R: Femoral head resurfacing for the treatment of osteonecrosis in the young patient. Clin Orthop Relat Res. 2003;417:93-101.
42. Beaule PE, Amstutz HC. Management of Ficat stage III and IV osteonecrosis of the hip. J Am Acad Orthop Surg. 2004;12:96-105.
43. Zhao D, Cui D, Wang B, et al. Treatment of early stage osteonecrosis of the femoral head with autologous implantation of bone marrow-derived and cultured mesenchymal stem cells. Bone 2012;50: 325–30.
44. Cenni E, Perut F, Dallari D, et al: In vitro evaluation of free-dried bone allografts combined with platelet rich plasma and human bone marrow stromal cells for tissue engineering. J Mater Sci Mater Med 2009;20:45-50.
45. Dallari D, Savarino L, Stagni C, et al.: Ehnanced tibial osteotomy healing with use of bone grafts supplemented with platelet ge or platelet gel and bone marrow stromal cells. J Bone Joint Surg Am 2007; 89:2413-20.
46. Dallari D, Fini M, Stagni C, et al: In vivo study on the healing of bone defects treated with bone marrow stromal cells, platelet rich plasma and freeze dried bone allografts, alone and in combination. J Orthop Res, 2006; 24:877-88.
47. Surgical dislocation of the adult hip a technique with full access to the femoral head and acetabulum without the risk of avascular necrosis. Ganz R, Gill TJ, Gautier E, Ganz K, Krügel N, Berlemann U.J Bone Joint Surg Br. 2001 Nov;83(8):1119-24.

CHAPTER 4

TREATMENT OF PSEUDOARTHROSIS

Luca Cevolani, Davide M. Donati, Benedetta Spazzoli, Stefano Pasini

Clinic III with prevalent oncological address
Rizzoli Orthopaedic Institute - Bologna

Consolidation delay and non-consolidation: definitions and differences

About two million long bone fractures are treated annually in the United States. According to Heppenstall [1], 5% of these results in a consolidation delay or even worse in pseudoarthrosis. The aggressive treatment implemented on some acute fractures has reduced the incidence but has increased paradoxically in other fractures, especially the tibia.

The difference between pseudoarthrosis and consolidation delay is predominantly to a degree. It is not possible to arbitrarily establish the time taken by a fracture to heal. We speak of consolidation delay when the consolidation does not proceed at the average speed for localization and fracture type (usually from 3 to 6 months).

A diagnosis of pseudoarthrosis is not real as long as there is no clinical or radiographic evidence of stopping the healing and consolidation process.

In 1986 as part of tests on bone healing devices, a group of experts from the Food and Drug Association (FDA) defined pseudoarthrosis as "established when a minimum of 9 months has passed since the trauma, and the fracture shows no visible signs of healing after 3 months". These criteria cannot be applied to all types of fractures. A diaphyseal fracture of a long bone cannot be considered pseudoarthrosis until at least 6 months after trauma because consolidation often takes longer, especially after local complications such as infections. On the contrary, a femoral neck fracture is defined as pseudoarthrosis after 3 months from the causal event.

Criteria for measuring effective bone consolidation

The consolidation of a fracture is a continuous and gradual process through which the process of bone regeneration restores the strength of a fractured bone. However, this represents an incomplete definition because bone regeneration can occur through various histological modalities (endosteal, periosteal, cortical). To extract from this variegated process a point of arrival represented by consolidation, a certain degree of arbitrariness must be accepted, which means converting a continuous variable into a category through the application of a threshold value. The choice of the continuous variable depends on what can be measured. Using an experimental model, biologists can directly measure the strength of bone consolidation, but clinicians must use an element that is representative of this, such as radiograms. The limits within which it is possible to define the successful union, as the objective of the study, must be established empirically. In addition, the appropriate definition of consolidation depends on the mode of regeneration in the situation under consideration. For example, in a diaphyseal fracture treated with rigid internal fixation and consolidation is expected through the union of the cortical, the objective includes the disappearance of any radiotransparency line visible in the cortical bone to radiograms and the absence of bone bridges for callus formation externally. However, fractures treated with an intramedullary nail consolidate largely through the external callus formation, and a consolidated fracture may still have the cortical fracture line clearly visible for a time. The appropriateness of the mechanical measurements also varies with the type of treatment. In a fracture of the tibial pylon treated with functional support, the degree of union can be measured through serial measurements of the flexural strength, which cannot be carried out in the same fracture treated with an intramedullary nail.

In addition, the consolidation delay is not just a problem of amount of time; nature offers different ways to lead to complete consolidation. A rapid endosteal reaction is undoubtedly the fastest mode based on an excellent intramedullary blood supply and good stability [2]. The periosteal reaction depends on the presence of an intact periosteum: it is a rapid process if the periosteum is detached for a short segment from the underlying bone. It is slower if the segment is of greater magnitude.

The slow process of endosteal repair, which can intervene after several months of delay when every periosteal response has shut down, is the reason why almost all failed consolidations will heal if left long enough in a plaster. However, if the periosteal response is finished and the endosteal pathway is no longer open, the situation is described as a non-union.

It can therefore be concluded that the consolidation process is defined as the reconstruction of the structure of a bone in which a fracture is present through endosteal bone regeneration, periosteal, or both. As already mentioned, the speed of healing that intervenes through periosteal regeneration depends on the extent of the damage to the surrounding soft tissues.

Consolidation delay is considered a process of forming a late intramedullary bone callus in which the periosteal response has ceased before the actual consolidation is achieved.

The lack of consolidation or pseudoarthrosis is a process of formation of scar tissue in which the share of endosteal and periosteal osteogenesis is zero since bone resorption has taken on more weight and is made evident by the lack of formation of new bone both for endosteal and periosteal production, with associated sclerosis of the bone marrow canal.

Classification of pseudoarthrosis

Pseudoarthrosis can be classified in numerous ways, both clinical and radiological.

Clinically they can be classified into infected and uninfected pseudoarthrosis.

Uninfected pseudoarthrosis

Uninfected pseudoarthrosis was described by Judet [4] and later by Weber and Cech [5] and were divided into two main types.

In the first, the ends of the stumps are hypervascularized or hypertrophic, that is, with biological reaction capacity. Studies on strontium-85 uptake in this group indicate a high blood supply at the ends of the stumps. Hypertrophic pseudoarthrosis are further divided into:

- *Pseudoarthrosis to "elephant's paw"*, these forms are hypertrophic and rich in callus. They result from unstable fixation, inadequate immobilization, or premature granting of the load in a reduced fracture with vital abutments.
- *Pseudoarthrosis to "horse hoof"*: these forms are on average hypertrophic and poor in callus. They are the result of a moderately unstable fixation with plates and screws. The ends of the stumps show a certain callus, insufficient for consolidation, and sometimes slight sclerosis.
- *Oligotrophic pseudoarthrosis:* they are not hypertrophic forms but show a good vascularization with absent callus. They are typically the result of large mobilizations of the fracture, distraction of the fragments, or internal fixation without adequate affixing.

In the second type, the ends of the stumps are avascular or atrophic, inert, and incapable of biological reaction. Studies on the incorporation of strontium-85 have indicated poor vascularization of the ends of the stumps in these forms.

Avascular pseudoarthrosis are further divided into:

- *"Torsion wedge" pseudoarthrosis* are forms characterized by an intermediate fragment with minimal or absent vascularization. This fragment is consolidated to one of the two stumps but not the other. This consolidation is typical of tibial fractures treated with plaques and screws.
- *Comminute pseudoarthrosis* are forms characterized by one or more necrotic interposed fragments. X-rays show no signs of callus. This condition is frequently evident following the rupture of plaques used in acute stabilization of the fracture.
- *Pseudoarthrosis with bone gap* are characterized by the loss of bone substance at the fracture level. The ends of the stumps are vital, but the consolidation of the defect is impossible with the passage of time, the extremities atrophy. This condition is evident after exposed fractures, sequestrecto-

my in the treatment of osteomyelitis, and resections for tumor.

- *Atrophic pseudoarthrosis* usually result from intermediate bone fragments not visualized and scar tissue devoid of osteogenetic potential left in situ. The ends of the stumps become osteoporotic and atrophic.

Pseudoarthrosis (not infected) finally, we must divide them in relation to: absence of bone defect; moderate bone defect; critical bone defect.

A "critical bone defect" can be defined as a bone defect that cannot resolve spontaneously unless supported by elements stimulating bone growth. In other words, a longitudinal defect greater than 2-2.5 times the diameter of a fractured bone cannot undergo spontaneous regeneration unless helped. According to the anatomical district concerned, the critical bone defect is classified differently: > 3 cm for the forearm; > 4 cm for the tibia; > 6 cm for the humerus and femur.

Infected pseudoarthrosis

Infected pseudoarthrosis is generally classified according to the extent of infection and synthesis stability. Cierny [5] provides a classification based on the local extent of the infection:

1. intramedullary osteomyelitis;
2. superficial osteomyelitis;
3. localized osteomyelitis;
4. diffuse osteomyelitis.

Each of these four types is further divided into 3 classes based on systemic characteristics:

- absence of impairment of the general state of health;
- presence of local or systemic impairment of fracture or wound healing;
- presence of high risk of perioperative complications.

Aetiology

Although the precise causes of consolidation delay and pseudoarthrosis are unknown, numerous systemic and local factors seem to contribute to their development.

Scientifically based research has shown that smoking and nicotine use have proven harmful to numerous biochemical processes involved in the process of bone consolidation, as nicotine negatively modifies arteriolar blood flow. Since the normal consolidation process is associated with inflammation and the synthesis of prostaglandins, nonsteroidal anti-inflammatory drugs (NSAIDs) that interfere with this process should theoretically interfere with the consolidation itself. However, this theory remains controversial [6].6

Dysmetabolic and endocrine diseases may also play a role in the process of bone consolidation. A recent study showed that patients with a lack of consolidation on an unknown basis had undiagnosed metabolic dysregulation, including hypothyroidism or vitamin D deficiency.

The patient's nutritional status also plays a significant role: chronic diseases or polytraumatized patients in a catabolic state potentially have impaired healing. Knowing all these risk factors is important to understand the normal consolidation process and its complications.

Patient-independent risk factors influencing bone consolidation are represented by the characteristics of the trauma - including the type of bone injury - the localization of the fracture, the state of the surrounding soft tissues, and the extent of bone loss. The localization of the fracture in a certain segment can alone represent a risk factor for non-consolidation. Sites such as the scaphoid, the metaphyseal region of the fifth metatarsal, or the body of the navicular bone of the tarsus receive a small blood supply and a fracture in these areas is believed to result in a potential impairment of the healing process. Similarly, exposed fractures have an altered consolidation secondary to soft tissue damage and an increased risk of infection.

The unstable synthesis of the fracture represents other variables that influence this process, the immobilization for an insufficient time, the positioning in distraction by traction, the synthesis of the plate and screws, and the radiant treatment prior to a fracture [2].

Treatment of consolidation delays

Non-surgical treatment

Birch was the first to use electricity to heal fractures clinically. In 1841 Hartshorne first reported the use of electricity in successfully treating missed tibial consolidations. Friedberg in 1971 used electrostimulation, and since then, many researchers have suggested its use in the treatment of this problem. These devices can use a direct current (DC), pulsating electromagnetic fields (PEMF) or combiners (CMF), an alternating current, or a capacitive coupling to provide electrostimulation at the site of a fracture. Electric fields were generated by an invasive technique in the bone, placing electrodes at the site of a healing fracture or, in a non-invasive manner, by means of a capacitive or inductive coupling.

Electric and electromagnetic fields are a biophysical technical form that regulates the synthesis of the extracellular matrix and can be useful in stimulating the repair of fractures and missed consolidations. These techniques have been used to treat recent fractures, osteotomies, spinal fusions, and late fractures.

Pharmacotherapy

Systemic treatment with vitamin D3 calcium has been shown to promote bone callus formation in both animal studies [7] and humans [8] within approximately 6 weeks after fracture. It has not yet been proven what the role of bisphosphonates is.

Capacitive coupling

Bassett developed this non-invasive technique, which requires the careful placement of two coils around the fracture site. The limb is immobilized in plaster, and the coils are placed on the plaster all around. Potentials of 1-10 V are applied at frequencies of 20-200 kHz, producing electric fields of about 1-100 mV/cm in the fabric. Capacitive coupling promotes bone healing of failed consolidations. In a study carried out to compare the healing rates obtained using a direct current, capacitive coupling, or bone graft, the findings suggested that the implantation of a graft gave lower percentages of consolidation if subsequent to the failure of a previous graft and that the capacitive coupling had a lower percentage of consolidation in the presence of atrophic pseudoarthrosis.

Direct electric current

Techniques using a direct electric current stimulate osteogenesis at the level of the cathode, with currents of 5-100 mA. Direct current can be supplied with semi-invasive or invasive methods. Friedenberg's semi-invasive technique consists of a power supply unit, which delivers a current of 20 mA, an anode consisting of a stainless steel grid applied to the skin, and a K-wire cathode of stainless steel. The cathode tip is inserted through the skin into the site of non-consolidation using a brilliance amplifier. The overall success rate, reported by Heppenstall in 50 missed forearm consolidations treated with 3 months of semi-invasive DC stimulation in the absence of diastasis and infection, was about 80%.

The invasive technique devised by Patterson involves a small operation to insert a generator that delivers a constant current of 20 mA. A platinum anode with titanium cathode is shaped in the shape of a propeller and placed through the site of non-consolidation. Zichner reported his successful experience with the invasive use of DC in 1981.

Inductive coupling

Electric fields can be produced in the bone using an inductive coupling (IC), with a variable external time or pulsed electromagnetic field. For the transport of current this technique uses a single or double coil, which is driven by an external field generator and which induces a secondary electric field in the bone.

Electromagnetic fields

CMF stimulators use an external coil with direct and alternating currents to produce both static and alternating magnetic fields. CMF units are available in many sizes and coil designs to fit various fracture sites. The patient may poorly tolerate the size and volume of CMF technology, but units are recommended for only 30 minutes of use per day. CMFs, a new type of biophysical stimulus, have been shown to stimulate the endogenous production of growth factors that regulate the healing process.

Exogenous electromagnetic fields are produced to promote the healing of fractures by invasive or non-invasive methods. It has been shown that the shear forces acting on a bone release electrical potentials on the osteocyte membrane, promoting fracture healing. The electromagnetic fields acting in vitro on osteoblasts stimulate the secretion of BMP-2 and 4, TGF-β and IGF-II, which, in turn, promote fracture healing. Pulsed electromagnetic stimulation has proven to be an effective modality, especially for the lack of hypertrophic consolidations, but it does not address the lower extremities' problems of instability, deformity, or asymmetry.

Heckman [9] reported a 64% cure of 149 patients using PEMFs, with a higher cure rate for the tibia than for the femur or humerus. As knowledge of the mechanisms of action expands, the specific energy needs of the fields are defined, and the range of treatable conditions is expanded. These conditions include nerve regeneration, wound healing, and diabetes. PEMFs potentiate angiogenesis primarily by stimulating the endothelial release of FGF-2 and inducing paracrine and autocrine modifications in the surrounding tissue. These findings suggest a potential role for PEMFs in therapeutic angiogenesis.

Pulsating ultrasound

Stimulation of bone growth with ultrasound consists of transmitting pulsed acoustic pressure waves of low density and other frequencies to accelerate the healing of recent fractures and promote the healing of late and missed consolidations, which are refractory to conventional treatment. The elements that transmit the pulse are also applied externally and consist of a battery power supply and a transduction head. The unit can be applied directly to the skin above the fracture site or, if necessary, by making a window into the plaster. Randomized trials have shown that using low-intensity pulsed ultrasound treatment can significantly reduce healing time for conservatively treated fractures. Treatment with an active ultrasound device also substantially reduced the incidence of tibia consolidation delays in smokers and non-smokers. Using an active ultrasound apparatus accelerates the healing of fractured cortical and spongy bone, substantially mitigates the healing retardant effects of cigarette smoke, accelerates the return to normal activities, and reduces long-term complications, such as delayed consolidation. It seems that ultrasound treatment does not give additional benefits after intramedullary nailing preceded by milling. Its use is gaining an increasingly wide consensus, and its ease of use makes it well tolerated by patients [2].

The current protocol requires the use of ultrasound for 20 minutes a day. It has been hypothesized that such treatment promotes consolidation by stimulating inflammation and bone regeneration mechanisms genes. Another theory holds that their effect is expressed by an increase in local blood flow through the dilation of capillaries and the stimulation of angiogenesis, thus increasing the flow of nutrients to the fracture site [2].

Surgical treatment

The type of surgical treatment varies depending on whether it is an infected or uninfected pseudoarthrosis. In the first case, it will be necessary to think first about solving the infectious picture since this is the necessary condition to allow the healing of pseudoarthrosis.

As for the uninfected forms, it will be of primary importance to identify the local and general risk factors that have determined the failure of bone repair [10]; only their intimate understanding will allow them to make the right corrections and restart the physiological healing mechanisms.

Recently the "*Diamond Concept*" (fig. 1) pointed out the different mechanical and biological appurtenances, the latter distinguished by cells, scaffolds, and growth factors that intervene in the healing process of fractures[11]. From a mechanical point of view, the spectrum of stability that considers the whole of bone and osteosynthesis implant must be restored. The stability spectrum interprets Wolff's law by indicating the need to modulate the rigidity of synthesis due to pseudoarthrosis's degree of intrinsic instability [12].

Internal fixation

Internal fixation techniques include the use of intramedullary nails or compression plates. The use of intramedullary nails allows to obtain a static fixation and can allow an early recovery of the load, although the boring of the intramedullary canal can cause the devascularization of the endosteal region for about 12 weeks [13].
In addition to nails, compression plates can provide a useful alternative [14–16]. Plaques lead to an increase in stability without, however, bringing an osteogenetic stimulus.

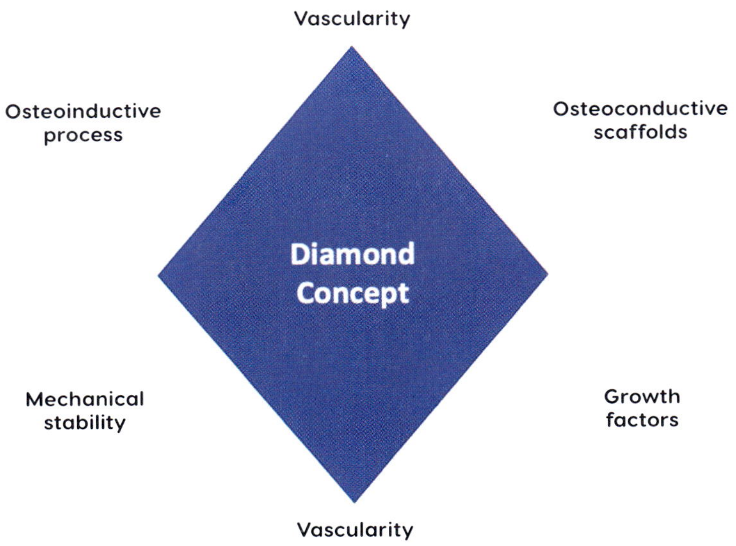

Figure 1 The model of the Diamond concept for the interaction of fracture healing processes.

External fixation

External fixation can be an alternative in the treatment of aseptic pseudoarthrosis, while it is the treatment of choice in septic pseudoarthrosis. In the latter case, it has many advantages (static synthesis of bone fragments, absence of implants, and respect for vascularization) and disadvantages (risk of infection of the pin tracts and the synthesis cannot be dynamized).

Treatment options

Considering the mechanical and biological aspects of the problem, there will be different indications of treatment depending on whether they are located at the diaphyseal, metaepiphysary, or epiphyseal level. It is, therefore, possible to hypothesize a treatment algorithm that takes into account all the above points:

Pseudoarthrosis without bone defect:

- Diaphyseal: intramedullary nailing (IEB) with or without application of bone growth factors (BMP);
- Metaepiphyseal: IEB or internal angular stability fixation (ASIF) with or without application of BMP;
- Epiphyseal: ASIF con or not application of BMP.

Pseudoarthrosis with minor bone defect:

- Diaphyseal: IEB in combination with BMP, scaffold with or without application of concentrated autologous mesenchymal cells (MSC);
- Metaepiphyseal: ASIF preferable to external fixation (EF) not in ligament axis in combination with BMP, scaffold with or without application of MSC;
- Epiphyseal: ASIF preferable EF in ligament takes in combination with BMP, scaffold with or without application of MSC.

Pseudoartrosi con critical bone defect:

- Diaphyseal: transport with EF in association with BMP at the docking point, or ASIF in combination with massive allograft soaked with MSC adjuvanted by BMP-7, ASIF in combination with scaffolds (xenon

+ allo) soaked with MSC adjuvanted by BMP-7;
- Metaepiphyseal: ASIF with massive grafting soaked with MSC adjuvanted by BMP;
- Epiphyseal: arthrodesis.

In case of infected pseudoarthrosis it becomes essential the removal of the means of synthesis, a suitable tissue surgical toilet, the complete removal of the infected pseudoarthrosis malacic tissue (en-block), the constitution of a new biological chamber obtainable through different methods:

- transport with EF in combination with BMP at docking point;
- antibiotic demineralized bone matrix graft in combination with scaffold + cast;
- antibiotic cement until normalization of inflammation indices and radiological investigations with EF, followed by removal of antibiotic cement, application of autograft adjuvanted by BMP, and osteosynthesis with ASIF [17–19].

Supportive biological therapies

Autologous bone grafting is still considered the treatment of choice because it naturally provides the basic components needed for skeletal repair. These include osteoinductive growth factors, the osteoconductive extracellular matrix, and osteogenic stem cells present among the cellular elements of the bone marrow.

Osteoinduction is defined as the process by which pluripotent mesenchymal stem cells are recruited from the surrounding host tissues, which then differentiate into osteoprogenitor cells destined to give life to the cellular elements forming the bone. This process is mediated by the growth factors coming from the graft. An osteoconductive material acts as a scaffold, supporting the interstitial growth of capillaries, perivascular tissues, and progenitor cells from the receiving tissue. This occurs according to an ordered sequence, determined by the three-dimensional structure of the graft, the local blood supply, and the biomechanical forces that insist on the graft and the surrounding tissues. In terms of grafting, an osteogenic material contains living cells capable

of differentiating into bone-forming elements.
Despite the effectiveness of autologous bone grafts, there are problems related to their use, such as the morbidity of donor sites, neurovascular lesions, and infection rates of 8-10% associated with graft removal. These problems have led to the search for alternative materials such as heterologous bone: however, despite its immediate availability, the risk of disease transmission, the reduced biological and mechanical properties compared to autologous bone, and the higher costs have limited its use.

Autologous bone grafts

Also known as autografts or autogenic grafts, they are parts of bone segments taken and implanted in the same individual that can consist of spongy, cortical bone (vascularized and non-vascularized grafts), and bone marrow. The incorporation of bone grafts occurs according to a sequence of events similar to that which occurs in the healing of fractures. Once implanted in the host, a hematoma forms on the periphery of the graft that releases bioactive molecules such as growth factors and proinflammatory cytokines. Mediators such as interleukin 1 (IL-1), IL-6, and tumor necrosis factor-alpha (TNF-α) are also secreted, which perform a chemotactic function on various bone marrow-derived cell types, including neutrophils, macrophages, and osteoclasts. These cells colonize the graft, initiating the resorptive phase of incorporation. Signal peptide molecules, such as platelet-derived growth factor (PDGF) and transformation-inducing growth factor β (TGF-β), exert a facilitative effect on the breakdown process by acting on the recruitment and differentiation of mesenchymal cells.
Once the inflammatory process has reduced, the formation of bone callus begins. A fibrovascular stroma develops where blood vessels and osteoprogenitor cells migrate to the graft. These pluripotent mesenchymal cells differentiate into osteoblasts that synthesize osteoids. At the same time, the graft undergoes partial necrosis, and osteoclasts continue to remove ne-

crotic bone debris with the release of additional biochemical mediators of repair from its extracellular matrix. Osteoblasts and lining endosteal cells, present on the surface of the graft, can survive transplantation and contribute to healing.

More likely, the most significant contribution offered by the graft is to constitute an osteoinductive and osteoconductive substrate. It guarantees the necessary physicochemical properties that make normal osteoblastic cells' adhesion, migration, division, and differentiation necessary for bone formation.

The remodeling process constitutes the last stage of the graft incorporation process with the formation of bone tissue with intertwined fibers that is then slowly transformed into the robust lamellar bone through the coordinated activity of osteoblasts and osteoclasts. The organization of the graft is also influenced by other events such as the quality of the tissues of the host site, including their vascularization, which affects the speed and extent of incorporation; an avascular bed poor in progenitor cells of the endothelium or connective tissue will be less able to respond to osteoinductive and osteoconductive signals starting from the graft. This can occur in patients undergoing radiation therapy previously or agents such as glucocorticoids and nicotine that impair cellular function. The presence of mechanical instability of the graft will determine the development of granulation tissue and fibrous tissue within the graft-host, preventing consolidation.

Autologous spongy bone grafts

Spongy bone, with its large surface area covered with lining cells and active osteoblasts, has the potential to induce more new bone than cortical grafts. Formation and resorption co-occur: osteoblasts lay osteoids on the surface of the necrotic bone, where osteoclasts slowly reabsorb dead trabeculae. The process of "creeping substitution" characterizes the last phase of transplantation: therefore, although the spongy bone provides little or no structural support, it is quickly incorporated and entirely replaced by the host bone and marrow within a year. These grafts are usually taken in small fragments from locations such as the iliac crest, the distal epiphysis of the radius, the large trochanter, and the proximal metaphyses of the tibia and distal femur.

Autologous cortical bone grafts

They are generally taken from the ribs, fibula, or bone shell of the ileum and can be implanted with or without their vascular peduncle. They possess mainly osteoconductive and little osteoinductive properties. The thickness of the cortical bone matrix limits the survival of osteocytes after transplantation, limiting its osteogenic properties. Due to the density of the cortical bone, the rate of revascularization is substantially slower, and this is observed more with non-vascularized grafts, in which vascular penetration is mainly the result of peripheral osteoclastic resorption and vascular invasion of the Volkmann and Havers channels.

Vascularized grafts are mostly independent of the host bed: the three primary sources of vascularized free grafts are the fibula with its peroneal vessels, the iliac crest with the deep iliac artery, and circumflex vein, and the ribs with the artery and posterior intercostal veins. Performed anastomosis of the vessels, 90% of osteocytes survive transplantation. As a result, the incorporation of the graft to the bone occurs more quickly without significant resorption and remodeling, so these grafts show greater resistance in the first 6 weeks after implantation. As with spongy bone, vascularized grafts require internal or external synthesis to have the necessary stability during the incorporation of the host bed.

Homologous bone grafts

It is an alternative to autologous bone since it avoids the morbidity of the donor site and its relative abundance allows it to adapt to the size of the loss of substance. There is a known relationship with the risk of transmission of diseases by the hematogenous route such that storage and sterilization procedures, such as freeze-drying or freezing, have been used to reduce the risk of transmission. Freeze-drying involves removing water from the fabric and packaging it under vacuum. Although this reduces immunogenicity, it has also been shown to reduce the mechanical integrity of the graft, thus affecting its ability to tolerate loads. In addition, freeze-drying weakens the graft's osteoinductive potential, causing cell death.

On the other hand, freezing reduces immunogenicity by decreasing the degradation of enzymes without altering mechanical properties. In general, the processes involved in incorporating homografts are much slower than those observed in non-vascularized autotransplants. This is partly related to the lack of vital donor cells that contribute to healing and the immune response during the inflammatory phase of incorporation. This deficiency of biological activity is manifested by incomplete revascularization, creeping substitution, and graft remodeling.

Histologically, mononuclear cells invade the graft and surround the newly formed vessels. These occlude, leading to rapid ischemic necrosis of the graft that remains in the host tissue and can be visible many years after implantation. Osteoinduction and osteoconduction are noticeably lacking. The biological nature of the receiving host bed is a critical factor in facilitating the incorporation of the graft. Cortical homografts, available as entire bone segments or cut as splints, confer mechanical stability and enhance consolidation. Their relative biological inertia limits the consolidation potential, but to improve this aspect, it is possible to insert autologous bone taken from the iliac crest to the homograft-host interface to provide the cells and osteoinductive proteins.

Autologous bone marrow

Connoly [20] was the first to bring back into clinical practice the use of autologous bone marrow in the treatment of tibia pseudoarthrosis. Injection of fresh marrow into bone substance leakage led to clinical and radiographic consolidation in 6 months. Garg also administered autologous bone marrow percutaneously to stimulate consolidation in 20 pseudoarthrosis of long bones; patients were banned from loading for 6 weeks after surgery then were granted until complete consolidation. In 17 out of 20 fractures, consolidation at 5 months was shown. These are all encouraging data to support the use of bone marrow in the treatment of fractures.

One of the downsides is the limited number of stem cells it contains. Muscher and coll. [21] noted that the mean prevalence of alkaline phosphatase-expressing colony-forming units (CFU-AP), a marker of osteoblast progenitors, is 55 per million nucleated cells. These values are undergoing a significant age-related decline for both men and women. They also noted that the volume of aspirate used for the grafting procedure could also influence the number of CFU-AP, which increases as the volume of aspirate increases, but at the same time also increases the degree of contamination of samples with peripheral blood. The researchers showed that an increase in volume from 1 ml to 4 ml causes an approximate decrease in CFU-AP of 50% and advise that the volume of aspirate taken from a single site does not exceed 2 ml.

Demineralized bone matrix

The demineralized bone marrow (DBM) bone matrix, produced by acid extraction of homologous bone, consists of tissue deprived of the mineral component. It is often mixed with conventional bone chips in the available preparations or associated with organic carriers. It has both "osteoconductive" and "osteoinductive" effects (fig. 2) thanks to the presence in the extracellular matrix of bone morphogenetic proteins (BMPs). It has been shown that this family of proteins, part of the TGF-β superfamily, is of primary importance in all bone reparative phenomena and therefore can stimulate the processes of angiogenesis and osteogenesis compellingly.

The implantation of DBM is followed by the formation of a hematoma and an inflammatory process characterized by the migration of polymorphonuclear into the implant within 18 hours. Mesenchymal cells differentiate into cartilage-producing chondro-

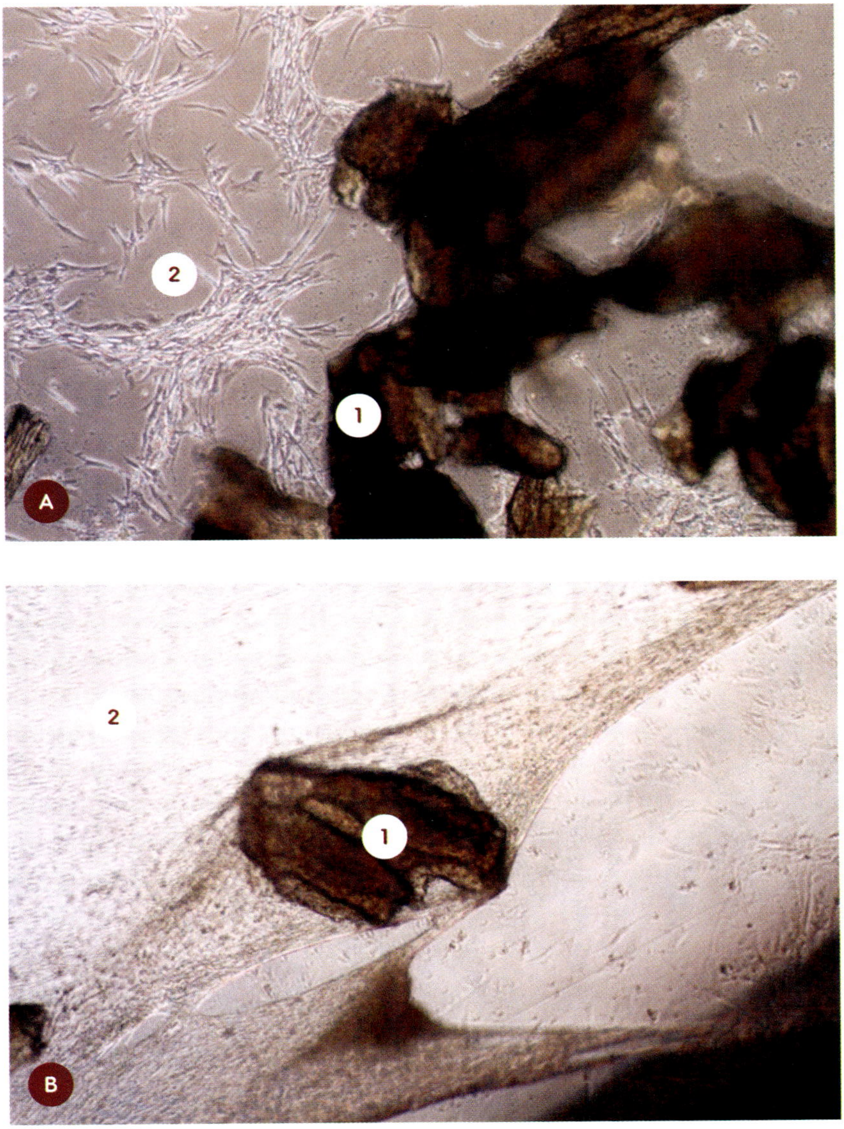

Figure 2 (A-B) Histological preparations in which DBM (1) and MSM (2) are found. Notice how cells tend to adhere and organize into colonies around DBM particles.

cytes on the fifth day. The cartilage undergoes mineralization and then is invaded by newly formed vessels on the tenth or twelfth day. The accompanying perivascular cells differentiate into osteoblasts, responsible for bone neoformation. The remodeling with resorption of all the implanted DBM takes place, which is thus replaced by the host bone.

There are different formulations of DBM based on the refinement of production techniques. They are available as freeze-dried powder, granules, gels, semi-solid paste, and splints. All show osteoconductive properties in animal studies, but no randomized controlled trials have been conducted in humans [2].

Bone substitutes: scaffold

Scaffolds are the necessary support to provide for the regrowth of bone tissue. It is a material intended to release, contain and form new tissue in vitro or to promote tissue repair in vivo. Porosity, architecture, and rate of degradation are important aspects of the material, which allow the growth of cells that drive the formation of bone tissue.

A bone substitute should meet three criteria:

- act as a scaffolding for osteoconduction;
- provide growth factors for osteoinduction;
- procure progenitor cells for osteogenesis.

Currently, available materials are phosphocalcium ceramics, calcium sulfate, bioactive glass, degradable polymers, recombinant human BMPs (OP-1 and BMP-2), and autologous bone marrow cells, meet only one of these criteria, and for this reason, there is a great interest in perfecting these materials.

Biomedical materials can be divided into three main types according to the response they provoke in the host tissue:

An inert material does not generate a response in the tissue.

A bioactive material is integrated by the surrounding tissues.

A degradable material reabsorbs and is incorporated into the surrounding tissue and can also dissolve entirely after a certain time.

The materials communicate with their

biological surroundings through their surface. The cellular response is then connected to the surface. After implantation, all materials are covered with whey proteins (fibronectin, vitronectin). The material's surface properties determine to what degree such a coating will be realized.

An ideal scaffold should also have the following characteristics:

- appropriate biocompatibility, not inducing any adverse reactions in the host tissue;
- appropriate degradation rate to correspond to the tissue regeneration process;
- adequate distribution of pore size to allow cells enough space to grow, access to nutrients and metabolites;
- high surface area to provide the cells with enough area to adhere;
- appropriate interaction with cells to promote their differentiation and growth;
- appropriate structural parameters to modulate cellular biosynthesis.

Phosphocalcium ceramics

Calcium phosphate ceramics are osteoconductive materials produced using a sintering process by which mineral salts are brought to temperatures of over 1000 ° C. Sintering reduces the amount of apatite carbonate, an unstable and weakly soluble form of hydroxyapatite. An ideal osteoconductive scaffolding should have an adequate three-dimensional structure that allows osseointegration and invasion of cells and blood vessels. It should also be biocompatible and biodegradable with biomechanical properties similar to the surrounding bone. Many of the ceramics used as bone-like grafts make osteoconduction possible. Despite this, their fragility and low resistance to tensile stress limit their use as grafting materials.

Hydroxyapatite (HA))

HA is a slow resorption compound derived from sea coral. A simple hydrothermal process converts coral into mechanically stable HA, with pores between 200 and 500 µm, a structure very similar to that of human transecular bone. Interpore (interpore International, Irvine, California, USA) is a coral HA and was the first bone substitute based on calcium phosphate, approved by the FDA. Hydroxyapatite is biocompatible and osteoconductive, but it is neither osteogenic nor osteoinductive and constitutes initial support with poor mechanical properties, which allow its use as a filling in the case of bone defects or to cover metal implants to improve its surface properties from the point of view of compatibility. Finally, it lacks connectivity between pores and is therefore fragile. Hydroxyapatite has been shown to be able to conduct the formation of bone tissue and form chemical bonds with bone without the interposition of a fibrous layer.

Tricalcium phosphate

TCP is a rapid resorption ceramic that undergoes a partial conversion to HA after implantation in the body. The HA is reabsorbed more slowly and remains in place for years.

Calcium sulphate

Calcium sulphate (hemihydrate), or Paris chalk, was first used in the early 1900s as a bone filler. It acts as an osteoconductive material that is completely reabsorbed while the newly formed bone reshapes itself and restores anatomical and structural features [2].

Polymers

Polymers are organic materials generated by controlled polymerization of individual molecules called monomers. Polymerization reactions can be multi-phase (condensation reactions) to obtain, for example, polyesters or radical addition reactions to obtain polystyrene or polyethylene.

Plants consisting of polymeric biomaterials have some advantages, some of which are: being easily produced in different forms (solids, films, viscoelastic materials, etc.); the possibility of modulation of chemical, physical and mechanical properties by forming copolymers or mixtures using different monomers in the same polymer; compared to metals they are not corroded; the density of polymers is similar to that of natural fabrics; given their similarity with the natural tissues (e.g., collagen) can be incorporated with other substances (e.g., heparin) by direct bond.

The disadvantages related to their use are instead: the low elastic modulus, especially for degradable polymers, which limits their use in applications where excellent resistance to the load is required; the very nature of polymerization that makes them biodegradable materials in the body; the difficulty in obtaining polymers that can be used as biomaterials without using additives, antioxidants, and plasticizers.

Polymers can have different structures: alternating, random, branched, block copolymers, they can form interpenetrated networks, or they can constitute compatible or incompatible mixtures according to the miscibility of the polymers.

Depending on their behavior after implantation or when in contact with biological fluids, biomedical polymers can be classified into non-degradable or biodegradable.

Typical non-degradable polymers are high molecular weight polyethylene, used in orthopedics; polymethylmethacrylate, polymerized in situ for bone cement or used for contact lenses; polydimethylsiloxane, used for soft tissues and intraocular lenses.

The polyesters used as a support are, for example, polylactic acid (PLA), polyglycolic acid (PGA), polycaprolactone (PCL), and their copolymers. Polylactic acid has a stereocenter that generates 2 possible isomers: a polymer consisting of L isomers is semi-crystalline, while D is more amorphous. Biodegradable polymers are used in Tissue Engineering, especially for the guided regeneration of bone and cartilage. The surface characteristics of the materials, together with the topography, play an important role in the adhesion of osteoblasts on the biomaterial. PCL is receiving significant attention in this field for its excellent physical properties, compatibility with tissues, and controlled degradation, which depends on porosity and copolymerization.

Phosphocalcium cement

Synthetic materials are now widely used, designed to summarize many of the characteristics necessary to perform the function of bone substitutes. Calcium phosphate cement (CPCs) can fill bone losses associated with recent fractures. To do this, it is necessary to use a combination of inorganic calcium and phosphate to obtain an injectable paste applied at the fracture site. Under physiological conditions, the material begins to harden in a few minutes, forming a mineral called dahllite, which is completed in about 12 hours, giving the cement compressive strength.

Regenerative medicine in the treatment of consolidation delays. How many cells are needed to form a bone callus?

The histological observation and the histomorphometric method proposed by Parfitt [22] and Frost [23] have helped the understanding of the functional and dynamic parameters associated with bone formation and subsequent tissue remodeling. In adult bone remodeling, these bone formation processes occur in the context of the multicellular basic units described by Frost [23]. Osteoblasts begin to secrete matrix in one day, and matrix synthesis increases over several days to a maximum of 1.5 μm per day for an area of about 150 μm^2 per osteoblast, resulting in a daily synthesis of about 225 μm^3 per osteoblast. Altogether, the synthesized matrix is about 6,000-9,000 μm^3 per osteoblast, about 3-5 times the cell volume. During the process of bone formation, some osteoblasts are incorporated into the new matrix as osteocytes, while others undergo apoptosis. The average lifespan of an osteoblast is just under 50 days, which is the time it takes to complete the bone formation process. Osteocyte density is higher in spongy bone (0.000047 osteocytes/μm^3) than in cortical bone (0.000026 osteocytes/μm^3) [21].

Rationale for using autologous bone marrow in the treatment of consolidation delays

A reduction in mesenchymal progenitor stem cells is noted in the tissues surrounding the consolidation delays. Bone marrow samples taken in adults from consolidation delay sites showed, after in vitro expansion, that the number of progenitor cells was very low compared to that taken from a tibia of healthy patients [24]. This difference can also be found in areas affected by infection, in sites involved in trauma or loss of substance, where scars are present, as well as a compromised vascularization frequently associated with consolidation delays [25]. This suggests that the local decrease in osteogenic cells may limit physiological tissue repair processes.

The relationship between the consolidation of a fracture and the activation of the bone marrow was first described by Ilizarov [26], who showed how the loss of 1% of blood induced an accelerated consolidation of an osteotomy rhyme in rats. The same study showed that, following significant blood loss, there was hematopoietic hyperactivity of the bone marrow of the iliac crest. This suggested a link between the hematopoietic activity of the iliac crest and osteogenesis around the osteotomy site. Experiments have also confirmed this phenomenon in rats and mice by Bab [27] and in rats by Lippiello [28]. A growth factor may give another hypothesis linking osteogenesis in an osteotomy outbreak and blood loss called osteopontin, whose secretion could be induced by blood loss. Lippiello's study also showed in the animal that when the bone marrow of the iliac crest contains more blood, the consolidation of a fracture is more rapid.

In recent years, an attempt has been made to increase the number of MSCs to be implanted using two distinct techniques: the sample's concentration and the laboratory's expansion.

Concentration

It involves using concentrated bone marrow immediately after the withdrawal in the operating room. Some studies have shown that bone marrow infiltration produces optimal effects when practiced early in the process of bone consolidation (not later than 6 months after the initial fracture) and is instead associated with modest results when practiced later (more than 18 months after fracture) [29].

This technique has many advantages, including a lower cost (compared to expansion), a single operating session in which the sampling and implantation take place, and the speed and simplicity of execution of the concentration procedure (although it differs according to the kit used). On the other hand, it does not allow us to know exactly how many MSCs are present before implanting them. It does not allow a selection of cells to be implanted and has lower efficacy than expanded cells (table 1).

Expansion in the laboratory

The use of expanded mesenchymal cells associated with a carrier biomaterial has long been considered a valid technique to replace autologous bone grafts [30,31]. However, there is no uniformity of thought about the adequacy on the origin of the different MSCs, the method of expansion, the reproducibility, the variability of the product obtained, and the quality of the final product.

Many studies, starting from the first work of Connoly et al. in 1991 [32], show how the number of implanted cells significantly increases the possibility of healing in consolidation delays [24, 33–45].

A considerable limit to the large-scale use of this method is given by the high cost of cell expansion (about € 20,000 for each sample), which must be added to the cost of using the operating room linked both to the withdrawal and subsequent implantation.

References

1. Heppenstall RB, Brighton CT, Esterhai JL, Muller G. Prognostic factors in nonunion of the tibia: an evaluation of 185 cases treated with constant direct current. J Trauma. settembre 1984;24(9):790–5.
2. Green R e. Adult Traumatology. Verduci Publisher; 2008.
3. Judet R. Treatment of Fractures Of The Femur Neck By Pedicule Graft. Acta Orthop Scand. 1 gennaio 1962;32(1–4):421–7.
4. Weber BG, Čech O. Pseudarthrosis: pathophysiology, biomechanics, therapy, results. New York: Grune & Stratton; 1976.
5. Cierny G, Mader JT, Penninck JJ. A clinical staging system for adult osteomyelitis. Clin Orthop. settembre 2003;(414):7–24.
6. Marsh D. Concepts of fracture union, delayed union, and nonunion. Clin Orthop. ottobre 1998;(355 Suppl):S22-30.

Table 1 Summary of literature papers describing the use of cells taken from the marrow for the treatment of consolidation delays. (LIPUS: low-intensity ultrasound; BM: bone marrow; BMC: concentrated bone marrow; NA: not applicable)

	Author/Years of publication	Number of patients	Localization	Average age (years)	Final result: healing (%)	Distance from I treatment	Note
1	Healey et al./1990 [46]	8	Femur (8)	27 (6-60)	5 (62,5)	4,95 (1-9)	Native BM in patients with bone resection for neoplasia and reconstruction with massive bone grafting
2	Connolly et al./1991 [32]	10	Tibia (10)	30 (18-82)	8 (80)	6,7 (5-10)	Native BM
3	Garg et al./1993 [47]	20	Tibia (15) Homer (3) Ulna (2)	35 (18-82)	17 (85)	5 (3-7)	Native BM
4	Sim et al./1993 [48]	11	Tibia (8) Femur (1) Other (2)	38 (19-62)	9 (81)	2,5 (1-5,75)	Native BM
5	Matsuda et al./1998 [49]	7	Femur (7)	53 (24-70)	4 (57)	on	Native BM
6	Siwach et al./2001 [50]	72	Tibia (42) Femur (8) Homer (12) Other(10)	41,2 (26-56)	68 (94)	on	Native BM
7	Wang et al./2001 [51]	56	Tibia (56)	na (19-72)	53 (94)	on	Native BM
8	Wilkins et al./2003 [52]	69	Tibia (36) Femur (16) Other (17)	42 (15-81)	61 (88)	8,1 (2-36)	Native BM and DBM
9	Goel et al./2005 [53]	20	Tibia (20)	37,5 (24-60)	15 (75)	3,5 (1,5-5,5)	Native BM
10	Hernigou et al./2005 [39]	60	Tibia (60)	40 (18-78)	53 (88)	3 (1-4)	BMC
11	Bhargava et al./2007 [54]	11	Tibia (11)	40,1 (24-51)	9 (81.8)	4,1 (1,7-6,4)	Native BM
12	Garnavos et al./2010 [55]	5	Homer (5)	na (30-75)	5 (100)	Na (12-20 weeks)	BMC
13	Singh et. Al./2013 [56]	12	Femur (3) Other (9)	45 (15-70)	10 (83)	4 (2,5-6)	Native BM
14	Kassem/2013 [57]	20	Tibia (13) Femur (5) Other (2)	42,3 (25-66)	19 (95)	2,95 (2-5)	Native BM
15	Sugaya et al./2013 [58]	17	Tibia (5) Femur (10) Other (2)	40,7 (22-80)	13 (76)	on	Native BM and LIPUS
16	Braly et al./2013 [59]	11	Tibia (11)	40,1 (24-51)	9 (81,8)	4,1 (1,7-6,4)	Native BM
17	Scaglione et al./2014 [60]	19	Tibia (7) Radio (3) Homer (3) Ulna (2) Femur (1) Metatarsus (1) Ulna (1) Fibula (1)	42,3 (20-73)	15 (78,9)	6.5 (na)	BMC e DBM
18	Barrena et al./2018 [36]	28	Femur (11) Tibia (13) Homer (4)	ON	26 (92%)	14,7 (2,1-36)	Expanded mesenchymal cells

7. Dickson K, Katzman S, Delgado E, Contreras D. Delayed unions and nonunions of open tibial fractures. Correlation with arteriography results. Clin Orthop. maggio 1994;(302):189–93.
8. Doetsch AM, Faber J, Lynnerup N, Wätjen I, Bliddal H, Danneskiold-Samsøe B. The effect of calcium and vitamin D3 supplementation on the healing of the proximal humerus fracture: a randomized placebo-controlled study. Calcif Tissue Int. settembre 2004;75(3):183–8.
9. Heckman JD, Ingram AJ, Loyd RD, Luck JV, Mayer PW. Nonunion treatment with pulsed electromagnetic fields. Clin Orthop. dicembre 1981;(161):58–66.
10. Calori GM, Albisetti W, Agus A, Iori S, Tagliabue L. Risk factors contributing to fracture non-unions. Injury. maggio 2007;38 Suppl 2:S11-18.
11. Giannoudis PV, Einhorn TA, Schmidmaier G, Marsh D. The diamond concept – open questions. Injury. settembre 2008;39, Supplement 2:S5–8.
12. Bergmann G, Duda G, Institut CBJW, Wolff J. Das Gesetz der Transformation der Knochen: Hirschwald, Berlin 1892 - Reprint 300 Seiten - Mit vier Nachworten und historischen Dokumente. 1., Auflage. Berlin: Pro Business; 2010. 300 pag.
13. Rhinelander FW. Tibial blood supply in relation to fracture healing. Clin Orthop. dicembre 1974;(105):34–81.
14. Di Maggio B, Grazioli A, Abate G, Italiano M. Our experience on the treatment of pseudoarthrosis of long bones with bone substitutes and PRP. Arch Ortop and Reumatol. December 1, 2013;124(1):12–4.
15. Zinghi G, Throne M, Rollo G. Pseudoarthrosis of long bones. Bologna: Timaeus; 2004. 280 p.
16. Siebert CH, Lehrbass-Sökeland KP, Rinke F, Hansis M. Compression plating of tibial fractures following primary external fixation. Arch Orthop Trauma Surg. 1997;116(6–7):390–5.
17. Klaue K, Knothe U, Anton C, Pfluger DH, Stoddart M, Masquelet AC, et al. Bone regeneration in long-bone defects: tissue compartmentalisation? In vivo study on bone defects in sheep. Injury. novembre 2009;40 Suppl 4:S95-102.
18. Giannoudis PV, Tzioupis C, Green J. Surgical techniques: how I do it? The Reamer/Irrigator/Aspirator (RIA) system. Injury. novembre 2009;40(11):1231–6.
19. Gilg MM, Liegl B, Wibmer C, Maurer-Ertl W, Leithner A. Central low-grade osteosarcoma with an unusual localization in the diaphysis of a 12-year old patient. Radiol Oncol. 21 maggio 2013;47(2):192–6.
20. Connolly JF, Shindell R. Percutaneous marrow injection for an ununited tibia. Nebr Med J. aprile 1986;71(4):105–7.
21. Muschler GF, Midura RJ, Nakamoto C. Practical Modeling Concepts for Connective Tissue Stem Cell and Progenitor Compartment Kinetics. J Biomed Biotechnol. 20 agosto 2003;2003(3):170–93.
22. Parfitt AM, Drezner MK, Glorieux FH, Kanis JA, Malluche H, Meunier PJ, et al. Bone histomorphometry: standardization of nomenclature, symbols, and units. Report of the ASBMR Histomorphometry

Nomenclature Committee. J Bone Miner Res Off J Am Soc Bone Miner Res. dicembre 1987;2(6):595–610.
23. Frost HM. The skeletal intermediary organization. Metab Bone Dis Relat Res. 1983;4(5):281–90.
24. Hernigou P, Beaujean F. [Bone marrow in patients with pseudarthrosis. A study of progenitor cells by in vitro cloning]. Rev Chir Orthopédique Réparatrice Appar Mot. 1997;83(1):33–40.
25. Brighton CT, Hunt RM. Early histological and ultrastructural changes in medullary fracture callus. J Bone Joint Surg Am. luglio 1991;73(6):832–47.
26. Ilizarov GA. The tension-stress effect on the genesis and growth of tissues: Part II. The influence of the rate and frequency of distraction. Clin Orthop. febbraio 1989;(239):263–85.
27. Bab I, Gazit D, Massarawa A, Sela J. Removal of tibial marrow induces increased formation of bone and cartilage in rat mandibular condyle. Calcif Tissue Int. settembre 1985;37(5):551–5.
28. Lippiello L, Chavda D, Connolly J. Colony-forming efficiency response of bone marrow stromal cells to acute blood loss. J Orthop Res Off Publ Orthop Res Soc. gennaio 1992;10(1):145–8.
29. Galois L, Bensoussan D, Diligent J, Pinzano A, Henrionnet C, Choufani E, et al. Autologous bone marrow graft and treatment of delayed and non-unions of long bones: technical aspects. Biomed Mater Eng. 2009;19(4–5):277–81.
30. Gómez-Barrena E, Rosset P, Müller I, Giordano R, Bunu C, Layrolle P, et al. Bone regeneration: stem cell therapies and clinical studies in orthopaedics and traumatology. J Cell Mol Med. giugno 2011;15(6):1266–86.
31. Gómez-Barrena E, Rosset P, Lozano D, Stanovici J, Ermthaller C, Gerbhard F. Bone fracture healing: Cell therapy in delayed unions and nonunions. Bone. 1 gennaio 2015;70:93–101.
32. Connolly JF, Guse R, Tiedeman J, Dehne R. Autologous marrow injection as a substitute for operative grafting of tibial nonunions. Clin Orthop. maggio 1991;(266):259–70.
33. Hernigou P, Mathieu G, Poignard A, Manicom O, Beaujean F, Rouard H. Percutaneous autologous bone-marrow grafting for nonunions. Surgical technique. J Bone Joint Surg Am. settembre 2006;88 Suppl 1 Pt 2:322–7.
34. Hernigou P, Pariat J, Queinnec S, Homma Y, Flouzat Lachaniette CH, Chevallier N, et al. Supercharging irradiated allografts with mesenchymal stem cells improves acetabular bone grafting in revision arthroplasty. Int Orthop. settembre 2014;38(9):1913–21.
35. Gómez-Barrena E, Padilla-Eguiluz NG, Avendaño-Solá C, Payares-Herrera C, Velasco-Iglesias A, Torres F, et al. A Multicentric, Open-Label, Randomized, Comparative Clinical Trial of Two Different Doses of Expanded hBM-MSCs Plus Biomaterial versus Iliac Crest Autograft, for Bone Healing in Nonunions after Long Bone Fractures: Study Protocol. Stem

Cells Int [Internet]. 22 febbraio 2018 [citato 27 agosto 2018];2018. Available at: https://www.ncbi.nlm.nih.gov/pmc/articles/PMC5842679/

36. Gómez-Barrena E, Rosset P, Gebhard F, Hernigou P, Baldini N, Rouard H, et al. Feasibility and safety of treating non-unions in tibia, femur and humerus with autologous, expanded, bone marrow-derived mesenchymal stromal cells associated with biphasic calcium phosphate biomaterials in a multicentric, non-comparative trial. Biomaterials [Internet]. 19 marzo 2018 [citato 27 agosto 2018]; Available at: http://www.sciencedirect.com/science/article/pii/S0142961218302059
37. Hernigou J, Schuind F. Smoking as a predictor of negative outcome in diaphyseal fracture healing. Int Orthop. maggio 2013;37(5):883–7.
38. Hernigou P, Poignard A, Manicom O, Mathieu G, Rouard H. The use of percutaneous autologous bone marrow transplantation in nonunion and avascular necrosis of bone. J Bone Joint Surg Br. luglio 2005;87(7):896–902.
39. Hernigou P, Poignard A, Beaujean F, Rouard H. Percutaneous autologous bone-marrow grafting for nonunions. Influence of the number and concentration of progenitor cells. J Bone Joint Surg Am. luglio 2005;87(7):1430–7.
40. Hernigou P. Bone transplantation and tissue engineering, part I. Mythology, miracles and fantasy: from Chimera to the Miracle of the Black Leg of Saints Cosmas and Damian and the cock of John Hunter. Int Orthop. dicembre 2014;38(12):2631–8.
41. Hernigou P. Bone transplantation and tissue engineering. Part II: bone graft and osteogenesis in the seventeenth, eighteenth and nineteenth centuries (Duhamel, Haller, Ollier and MacEwen). Int Orthop. 15 novembre 2014;39(1):193–204.
42. Hernigou P. Bone transplantation and tissue engineering, part IV. Mesenchymal stem cells: history in orthopedic surgery from Cohnheim and Goujon to the Nobel Prize of Yamanaka. Int Orthop. 7 marzo 2015;39(4):807–17.
43. Hernigou P, Beaujean F. Abnormalities in the Bone Marrow of the Iliac Crest in Patients Who Have Osteonecrosis Secondary to Corticosteroid Therapy or Alcohol Abuse*. J Bone Jt Surg. 1 luglio 1997;79(7):1047–53.
44. Hernigou P. Bone transplantation and tissue engineering, part III: allografts, bone grafting and bone banking in the twentieth century. Int Orthop. 21 gennaio 2015;39(3):577–87.
45. Homma Y, Zimmermann G, Hernigou P. Cellular therapies for the treatment of non-union: The past, present and future. Injury. gennaio 2013;44, Supplement 1:S46–9.
46. Healey JH, Zimmerman PA, McDonnell JM, Lane JM. Percutaneous bone marrow grafting of delayed union and nonunion in cancer patients. Clin Orthop. luglio 1990;(256):280–5.
47. Garg NK, Gaur S, Sharma S. Percutaneous autogenous bone marrow grafting in 20 cases of ununited fracture. Acta Orthop

Scand. dicembre 1993;64(6):671–2.
48. Sim R, Liang TS, Tay BK. Autologous marrow injection in the treatment of delayed and non-union in long bones. Singapore Med J. ottobre 1993;34(5):412–7.
49. Matsuda Y, Sakayama K, Okumura H, Kawatani Y, Mashima N, Shibata T. Percutaneous autologous bone marrow transplantation for nonunion of the femur. Nihon Geka Hokan Arch Für Jpn Chir. 1 marzo 1998;67(1):10–7.
50. Siwach RC, Sangwan SS, Singh R, Goel A. Role of percutaneous bone marrow grafting in delayed unions, non-unions and poor regenerates. Indian J Med Sci. giugno 2001;55(6):326–36.
51. Wang L, Li WS, Zhang QS. [Autogenous bone marrow graft for the management of nonunion of tibia]. Zhongguo Xiu Fu Chong Jian Wai Ke Za Zhi Zhongguo Xiufu Chongjian Waike Zazhi Chin J Reparative Reconstr Surg. gennaio 2001;15(1):24–5.
52. Wilkins RM, Kelly CM. The effect of allomatrix injectable putty on the outcome of long bone applications. Orthopedics. maggio 2003;26(5 Suppl):s567-570.
53. Goel A, Sangwan SS, Siwach RC, Ali AM. Percutaneous bone marrow grafting for the treatment of tibial non-union. Injury. gennaio 2005;36(1):203–6.
54. Bhargava R, Sankhla S, Gupta A, Changani R, Gagal K. Percutaneous autologus bone marrow injection in the treatment of delayed or nonunion. Indian J Orthop. gennaio 2007;41(1):67–71.
55. Garnavos C, Mouzopoulos G, Morakis E. Fixed intramedullary nailing and percutaneous autologous concentrated bone-marrow grafting can promote bone healing in humeral-shaft fractures with delayed union. Injury. giugno 2010;41(6):563–7.
56. Singh AK, Shetty S, Saraswathy JJ, Sinha A. Percutaneous autologous bone marrow injections for delayed or non-union of bones. J Orthop Surg Hong Kong. aprile 2013;21(1):60–4.
57. Kassem MS. Percutaneous autogenous bone marrow injection for delayed union or non union of fractures after internal fixation. Acta Orthop Belg. dicembre 2013;79(6):711–7.
58. Sugaya H, Mishima H, Aoto K, Li M, Shimizu Y, Yoshioka T, et al. Percutaneous autologous concentrated bone marrow grafting in the treatment for nonunion. Eur J Orthop Surg Traumatol Orthopédie Traumatol. luglio 2014;24(5):671–8.
59. Braly HL, O'Connor DP, Brinker MR. Percutaneous Autologous Bone Marrow Injection in the Treatment of Distal Meta-diaphyseal Tibial Nonunions and Delayed Unions: J Orthop Trauma. settembre 2013;27(9):527–33.
60. Scaglione M, Fabbri L, Dell'Omo D, Gambini F, Guido G. Long bone nonunions treated with autologous concentrated bone marrow-derived cells combined with dried bone allograft. Musculoskelet Surg. agosto 2014;98(2):101–6.

CHAPTER 5

REGENERATIVE THERAPY OF THE MUSCULOSKELETAL SYSTEM: APPLICATIONS OF PLATELET- RICH PLASMA

Giuseppe Filardo[1,2,3], Angelo Boffa[4], Luca Andriolo[4], Alessandro Di Martino[4]

1) Applied and Translational Research (ATR) center, IRCCS Rizzoli Orthopaedic Institute, Bologna, Italy;

2) Orthopaedic and Traumatology Unit, Ospedale Regionale di Lugano, EOC, Lugano, Switzerland (CH);

3) USI-Università della Svizzera Italiana, Faculty of Biomedical Sciences, Lugano, Switzerland (CH);

4) Orthopaedic and Traumatological Clinic 2, IRCCS Rizzoli Orthopaedic Institute, Bologna, Italy;

Abstract

In recent years the Platelet-Rich Plasma (PRP) has achieved great success in clinical practice, thanks to its safety, low costs, and simple preparation technique, which allows to exploit its biologically active content. The high concentrations of growth factors, cytokines, and other bioactive molecules released by platelets make this product suitable for clinical conditions requiring prompt and adequate healing support. PRP has been used in tendon diseases, where promising pre-clinical results have not been confirmed in clinical practice, with even harmful results in some studies on the Achilles tendon. At the same time, its benefits in cuff tendinopathies, epicondylitis, and patellar tendinopathy remain controversial. In acute muscle injuries, PRP has been applied to promote the regeneration of muscle fibers at the expense of scar tissue deposition, but even in this area, it has not shown great clinical benefits, if not a minimal reduction in the time of return to sport. The Platelet-rich plasma has been used as an “augmentation” in several surgical techniques, obtaining good results in association with microfractures or scaffolds for the treatment of focal cartilage lesions, while it has not added particular benefits to anterior cruciate ligament reconstruction techniques. The most significant evidence on PRP is instead for its intra-articular use in the treatment of osteoarthritis, especially knee. PRP seems to promote a better joint environment, favoring the restoration of a homeostatic balance in joints affected by degenerative processes. Numerous pre-clinical and clinical studies have described the efficacy and safety of intra-articular infiltration of PRP in patients with knee osteoarthritis, and recent meta-analyses have reported the superiority of this product over saline corticosteroids hyaluronic acid. Despite this, the most suitable type of PRP remains debated, with different preparation methods available that can give products with different compositions and properties. Therefore, it will be crucial in the future to better characterize the PRP and determine the aspects that can improve its benefits or affect its effectiveness. It will also be necessary to investigate its role in the various orthopedic pathologies with large and high-level studies to define the potential and limits of this biological treatment.

Introduction

Almost twenty years have passed since the first Platelet-Rich Plasma (PRP) applications in clinical practice. Since then, the interest in this organic product has grown dramatically, with thousands of articles that have studied its characteristics, biological rationale, safety, and clinical benefits in the treatment of various diseases. The success of PRP is linked to high concentrations of growth factors, cytokines, and other molecules stored in α-platelet granules. These bioactive molecules make PRP able to promote tissue repair and influence the reactivity of cells in inflammatory processes. PRP, therefore, represents an attractive biological approach for those clinical conditions that require support for rapid and adequate healing, being useful and effective, especially for tissues with low healing potential. Thanks to the safety, low costs, and simple preparation technique to obtain its biologically active content (fig. 1), PRP is gaining wide use in clinical practice, showing promising results in different fields of medicine, from dermatology to surgical disciplines. In orthopedics, PRP has had a universal application, with the greatest uses in the field of tendinopathies, muscle injuries, as "augmentation" to surgical techniques, but above all in the infiltrative treatment of cartilaginous degeneration and osteoarthritis (OA).

Platelet-rich plasma in muscle-tendon lesions

In pre-clinical models, PRP has achieved promising effects on tenocytes and the extra-cellular tendon matrix. Several pre-clinical studies have shown that it is able to increase collagen expression, tenocyte prolif-

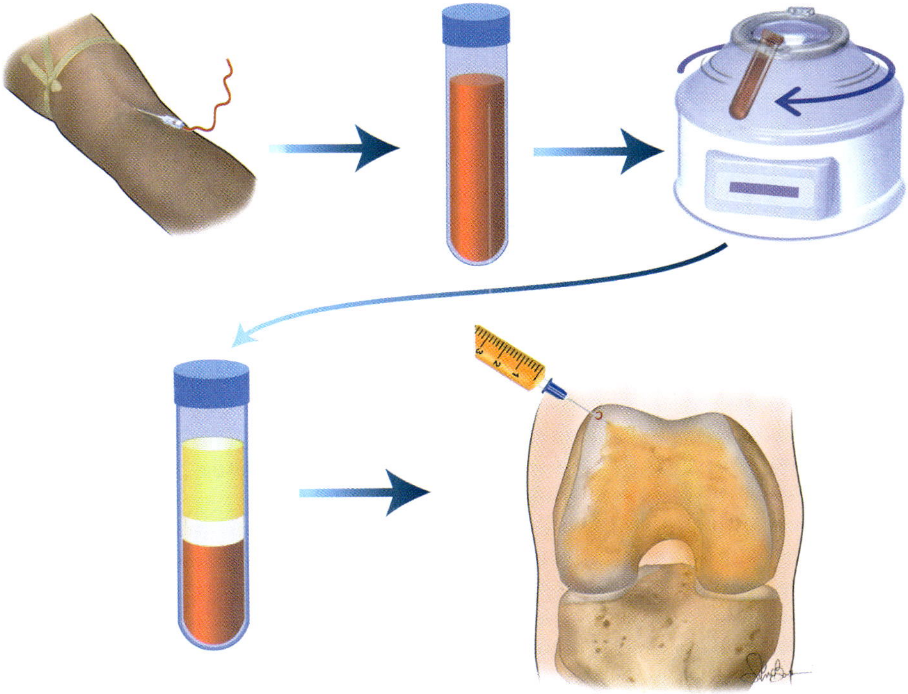

Figure 1 Peripheral venous blood sampling is performed. Through a centrifuge, the blood components are separated, obtaining three layers: plasma (55%), "buffy coat" with leukocytes and platelets (<1%), and erythrocytes (45%). Erythrocytes and platelet-poor plasma are eliminated to obtain platelet-rich plasma (with or without leukocytes) – PRP, ready to be used.

eration, and the expression of growth factors such as Transforming Growth Factor beta (TGF-β), Platelet-Derived Growth Factor (PDGF), and the Vascular Endothelial Growth Factor (VEGF). In this way, PRP could theoretically promote early tendon healing, increasing the repair rate and resistance to load and traction [1]. However, most pre-clinical studies have analyzed the effects of PRP on small animal models and acute tendon injury models, although the main clinical applications of PRP are actually on chronic tendinopathies. A recent systematic review of the literature analyzed 92 clinical trials that evaluated PRP's effectiveness in treating tendon diseases [2].

Regarding the Achilles tendon, PRP has been used for the conservative treatment of chronic tendinopathy or as adjuvant therapy to treat acute tendon ruptures. PRP has not shown a clear superiority over saline or rehabilitation in these pathologies, and in some cases, it has even proved harmful to tissue healing [3-5]. Clinical studies on PRP use for rotator cuff and elbow tendinopathies (epicondylitis and epitrocleitis) have reported controversial results, without highlighting a clear efficacy of PRP against other treatment methods such as unmanipulated blood injections, cortisone, local anesthetics, or laser therapy [6-8]. The use of PRP as a conservative treatment of patellar tendinopathy has suggested promising results, although the number of high-level studies is really low [9]. In addition, a recent single-blind randomized controlled trial (RCT) evaluated 57 patients with patellar tendinopathy treated with a single ultrasound-guided injection of leukocyte-rich PRP or leukocyte- or saline-poor PRP [10]. Surprisingly, the 3 treatment groups achieved significant clinical improvements up to 52 weeks after injection, but no significant difference was found between the 3 groups.

PRP has also been frequently used to treat acute muscle injuries. Following a muscle injury, two opposite biological phenomena occur: the regeneration of destroyed muscle fibers and the production of scar tissue [11].Platelet activation and the release of growth factors can play a key role in the early post-injury phase, as they orchestrate the healing process before the onset of the fibrosis phase (approximately 2-3 weeks after injury), which can be detrimental to subsequent muscle function [12]. The elevated concentrations of platelets and growth factors contained in PRP could thus promote a better healing response of muscle tissue, favoring the regeneration of muscle fibers rather than the deposition of scar tissue. A recent meta-analysis analyzed 6 RCTs (374 patients) that evaluated the effectiveness of PRP versus saline or physical therapy for the treatment of acute muscle injuries [13]. Patients treated with PRP had a significantly shorter time to return to sport than patients in the control groups, with an average difference of 7 days. However, this difference was canceled when only double-blind studies or only hamstrings studies were considered. There were no significant differences between the PRP and control groups regarding the risk of recurrence and post-treatment complications, muscle strength, joint range of motion (ROM), muscle function, and imaging. Therefore, despite its promising biological rationale, the efficacy of PRP injections in the treatment of acute muscle injuries has not been confirmed by studies of a high level of evidence.

PRP in surgical procedures

The healing potential of PRP has also been exploited in association with several surgical procedures. Biological “augmentation” with PRP was used to optimize the quality of the repair tissue, and consequently, the clinical results obtained by the microfracture technique in the treatment of focal cartilaginous lesions. The fibrocartilaginous tissue obtained with microfractures has, in fact, lower biological and biomechanical properties than hyaline cartilage, undergoing an early deterioration over time that is reflected in the long-term clinical results [14]. The rationale for using PRP in addition to this technique lies in the release of growth factors by platelets. They could play a crucial role in improving the quality of chondrogenesis by promoting matrix deposition and proteoglycan synthesis and promoting chondrogenic differentiation of mesenchymal stromal cells (MSCs) from the bone marrow of the subchondral bone [15, 16]. Pre-clinical studies have confirmed the benefits of adding PRP to microfractures, demonstrating better macroscopic, histological, and biomechanical properties in animal models treated with the addition of PRP compared to those treated with microfractures alone. However, the best results were found when PRP was applied directly into the cartilage defect during surgery, in the form of a gel, rather than following post-operative intra-articular infiltration [17, 18]. Promising pre-clinical results has led to PRP's use as an "augmentation" of microfractures also in clinical practice. A recent meta-analysis analyzed 7 clinical trials (234 patients) that compared the effectiveness of PRP in addition to microfractures compared to the surgical technique alone in patients with cartilage lesions of the knee or ankle [19]. Analysis of all scores at 12 and 24 months showed better clinical outcomes in patients treated with the addition of PRP, both for the knee and ankle, compared to patients treated with microfractures alone. However, the improvement offered by PRP did not reach the "Minimal Clinically Important Difference" (MCID); therefore, it was not perceptible by patients.

PRP has also been used as an augmentation technique to improve the results of procedures based on scaffolds for the treatment of cartilage defects. In particular, the scaffold can be impregnated with PRP before being implanted in the cartilage defect, with the aim of acquiring localized growth factors capable of facilitating the infiltration, proliferation, and differentiation of MSCs [20]. Several pre-clinical studies have investigated the role of adding PRP to scaffolds but found mixed results. On the one hand, some authors reported better histological and biomechanical results when the scaffold was implanted after the addition of PRP rather than alone [21, 22]. On the other hand, some authors reported worse results with the addition of PRP to the scaffold [23]. In clinical practice, PRP has been combined with different types of scaffolds, although studies in this regard are still few and of low level of evidence [24]. A clinical study evaluated the "augmentation" of PRP in autologous matrix-induced chondrogenesis (AMIC), a technique in which a type I/III porcine collagen membrane is used to cover the cartilage defect after microfractures. AMIC has been used with PRP to treat small numbers of patients with osteochondral lesions, including patella, reporting promising clinical results at 24 months of follow-up [25]. PRP has also been used in addition to new synthetic matrices, such as polyglycolic-hyaluronane acid (PGA-HA) implants, showing satisfactory clinical results of up to 24 months of follow-up in patients with focal chondral knee defects [20]. Histological evaluation in some of these patients documented a repair tissue similar to hyaline cartilage, i.e., rich in cells with chondrocyte morphology, proteoglycans, and type II collagen. PRP has also been used in combination with MSCs of bone marrow origin for the "augmentation" of hyaluronic acid or porcini collagen membrane, reporting positive results in the treatment of osteochondral lesions of both the knee and ankle [26, 27]. This technique, which can be performed in a single surgical step, has also demonstrated clinical results comparable to those obtained by the implantation of autologous chondrocytes (ACI), a technique that requires two surgical steps [28].

Numerous studies have evaluated the efficacy of PRP in anterior cruciate ligament reconstructive surgery (ACL), exploiting its many effects, including anabolic stimulation towards cells, increased extracellular matrix deposition, reduction of pro-apoptotic signals, and anti-inflammatory effect in the joint environment [29]. A systematic review of the literature analyzed 34 pre-clinical and clinical studies that evaluated the efficacy of PRP as an adjuvant of ACL surgery [30]. Pre-clinical evidence has found that PRP can improve the healing potential of tendon grafting in terms of histological and biomechanical performance. However, clinical trials have not confirmed the same results. Some of them have suggested that PRP could promote the healing of the donor site in case of reconstruction of the ACL with patellar tendon grafting and contribute positively to the maturation of the graft over time. On the other hand, most of the articles have not reported beneficial effects of PRP in terms of integration of the graft in the bone tunnel, but above all, a superiority of the functional results for short-term evaluation has not been demonstrated.

Platelet-rich plasma in osteoarthritis

Most studies related to PRP in orthopedics are focused on OA, especially knee OA. The growth factors released by platelets seem to be able to promote a better joint environment, favoring the restoration of a homeostatic balance in joints with cartilage degeneration [31]. Numerous in vitro studies have described the beneficial effects of PRP on chondrocytes and synoviocytes, and meniscal cells [31, 32]. In addition, PRP has shown an analgesic effect, probably through modulation of cannabinoid receptors in chondrocytes [33]. In addition to the biological rationale, current pre-clinical evidence further supports the role of PRP in modulating the intra-articular environment through anti-inflammatory action. In particular, after an initial pro-inflammatory activity, synoviocytes stimulation to release metalloproteinases and cytokines, a subsequent phase of modulation and reduction of the inflammatory response has been demonstrated, counteracting the chemotaxis of monocytic cells and decreasing pro-inflammatory cytokines [34]. Based on this evidence, it is important to emphasize that the main effect of PRP may not be a direct promotion of tissue regeneration. Still, it could act through its different bioactive molecules influencing the homeostasis of joint tissues, slowing down the inflammatory, catabolic and degenerative process, thus offering clinical benefits in terms of symptom relief and functional improvement.

These characteristics have led to the widespread use of PRP in clinical practice as an infiltrative therapy in osteoarthritis patients. PRP infiltrations have been shown to be safe and effective in reducing painful symptoms and improving joint function and quality of life in patients with knee OA. However, the benefits of PRP would seem to be valid, especially in younger patients with a low degree of joint degeneration [35, 36]. The efficacy of PRP would appear to be "time-dependent," with numerous studies reporting the effectiveness of up to 12 months after treatment [31]. Some evidence suggests that the clinical improvement provided by PRP may be felt by some patients even beyond 24 months, resulting in a gradual reduction over time [37]. Despite the significant placebo effect attributed to intra-articular infiltrations, particularly when it comes to a new biological product such as PRP [38], a recent meta-analysis focusing on 34 RCTs reported that infiltrations of PRP provided a statistically and clinically significant improvement in patients with knee OA compared to saline infiltration at 12-month follow-up, without increasing the risk of adverse events [39]. In addition, PRP injections provided better results than other commonly used injection strategies such as corticosteroids or hyaluronic acid. This benefit is increased over time, not being significant in previous follow-ups but becoming clinically significant after 6-12 months. However, although substantial (higher than MCID), the improvement remained partial and supported by a low level of evidence [39]. The partial improvement provided by PRP has also recently been shown in a study carried out on a cohort of sports patients with OA or degeneration of knee cartilage [40]. In this young population (mean age 41 years), infiltrative treatment with PRP provided good clinical results, although the results were less satisfactory in return to sport. In fact, only half of the patients analyzed had achieved a level of sport comparable to that present before the onset of symptoms.

Despite a large number of clinical studies on the intra-articular use of PRP, this product is not yet recommended by leading international companies for the treatment of knee OA [41-43]. This is probably due to the lack of standardization of the PRP used in clinical practice, producing different products and consequently still controversial results. In particular, the most suitable type of concentrate remains debated, with different preparation methods available for PRP that can give products with different composition and properties, with varying characteristics in terms of platelet and leukocyte content, the volume of whole blood collected, storage procedures, platelet activation and formation of a fibrin matrix [44]. All this makes it very complex to merge and analyze the clinical results of different studies and thus acquire a complete understanding of the real benefits of this biological approach. Further studies will need to investigate these aspects better to understand PRP's potential and limitations for OA treatment.

Conclusions

The results of PRP in the various orthopaedic pathologies are still controversial, and the evidence is based on a low number of high-level studies. Therefore, PRP will have to be further studied in the future, investigating its role in the different orthopedic pathologies in large high-level studies, explicitly defining the potential and limits of this biological treatment. It will be essential to characterize the PRP better and determine the aspects that can enhance its benefits or affect its effectiveness. In addition, it will be important to identify which patients may benefit most from treatment with PRP, determining the factors that influence their response to this biological approach, moving from baseline clinical features to biomarker profiles in serum or synovial fluid. Only after a correct characterization of the type of PRP used and the presence of solid data to support its safety and efficacy will it be possible to further extend this promising biological approach from clinical trials to clinical practice for the treatment of orthopedic pathologies.

References

1. Baksh N, Hannon CP, Murawski CD, Smyth NA, Kennedy JG. Platelet-rich plasma in tendon models: a systematic review of basic science literature. Arthroscopy : the journal of arthroscopic & related surgery : official publication of the Arthroscopy Association of North America and the International Arthroscopy Association. 2013 Mar;29(3):596-607.
2. Filardo G, Di Matteo B, Kon E, Merli G,

Marcacci M. Platelet-rich plasma in tendon-related disorders: results and indications. Knee surgery, sports traumatology, arthroscopy : official journal of the ESSKA. 2018 Jul;26(7):1984-99.

3. Krogh TP, Ellingsen T, Christensen R, Jensen P, Fredberg U. Ultrasound-Guided Injection Therapy of Achilles Tendinopathy With Platelet-Rich Plasma or Saline: A Randomized, Blinded, Placebo-Controlled Trial. The American journal of sports medicine. 2016 Aug;44(8):1990-7.
4. Kearney RS, Parsons N, Costa ML. Achilles tendinopathy management: A pilot randomised controlled trial comparing platelet-richplasma injection with an eccentric loading programme. Bone & joint research. 2013;2(10):227-32.
5. Schepull T, Kvist J, Norrman H, Trinks M, Berlin G, Aspenberg P. Autologous platelets have no effect on the healing of human achilles tendon ruptures: a randomized single-blind study. The American journal of sports medicine. 2011 Jan;39(1):38-47.
6. Palacio EP, Schiavetti RR, Kanematsu M, Ikeda TM, Mizobuchi RR, Galbiatti JA. Effects of platelet-rich plasma on lateral epicondylitis of the elbow: prospective randomized controlled trial. Revista brasileira de ortopedia. 2016 Jan-Feb;51(1):90-5.
7. Mishra AK, Skrepnik NV, Edwards SG, Jones GL, Sampson S, Vermillion DA, et al. Efficacy of platelet-rich plasma for chronic tennis elbow: a double-blind, prospective, multicenter, randomized controlled trial of 230 patients. The American journal of sports medicine. 2014 Feb;42(2):463-71.
8. Tetschke E, Rudolf M, Lohmann CH, Starke C. Autologous proliferative therapies in recalcitrant lateral epicondylitis. American journal of physical medicine & rehabilitation. 2015 Sep;94(9):696-706.
9. Vetrano M, Castorina A, Vulpiani MC, Baldini R, Pavan A, Ferretti A. Platelet-rich plasma versus focused shock waves in the treatment of jumper's knee in athletes. The American journal of sports medicine. 2013 Apr;41(4):795-803.
10. Scott A, LaPrade RF, Harmon KG, Filardo G, Kon E, Della Villa S, et al. Platelet-Rich Plasma for Patellar Tendinopathy: A Randomized Controlled Trial of Leukocyte-Rich PRP or Leukocyte-Poor PRP Versus Saline. The American journal of sports medicine. 2019 Jun;47(7):1654-61.
11. Drezner JA. Practical management: hamstring muscle injuries. Clinical journal of sport medicine : official journal of the Canadian Academy of Sport Medicine. 2003 Jan;13(1):48-52.
12. Huard J, Li Y, Fu FH. Muscle injuries and repair: current trends in research. The Journal of bone and joint surgery American volume. 2002 May;84(5):822-32.
13. Grassi A, Napoli F, Romandini I, Samuelsson K, Zaffagnini S, Candrian C, et al. Is Platelet-Rich Plasma (PRP) Effective in the Treatment of Acute Muscle Injuries? A Systematic Review and Meta-Analysis. Sports Med. 2018 Apr;48(4):971-89.

14. Case JM, Scopp JM. Treatment of Articular Cartilage Defects of the Knee With Microfracture and Enhanced Microfracture Techniques. Sports medicine and arthroscopy review. 2016 Jun;24(2):63-8.
15. Noth U, Rackwitz L, Heymer A, Weber M, Baumann B, Steinert A, et al. Chondrogenic differentiation of human mesenchymal stem cells in collagen type I hydrogels. Journal of biomedical materials research Part A. 2007 Dec 1;83(3):626-35.
16. Schmidt MB, Chen EH, Lynch SE. A review of the effects of insulin-like growth factor and platelet derived growth factor on in vivo cartilage healing and repair. Osteoarthritis and cartilage. 2006 May;14(5):403-12.
17. Milano G, Deriu L, Sanna Passino E, Masala G, Manunta A, Postacchini R, et al. Repeated platelet concentrate injections enhance reparative response of microfractures in the treatment of chondral defects of the knee: an experimental study in an animal model. Arthroscopy : the journal of arthroscopic & related surgery : official publication of the Arthroscopy Association of North America and the International Arthroscopy Association. 2012 May;28(5):688-701.
18. Milano G, Sanna Passino E, Deriu L, Careddu G, Manunta L, Manunta A, et al. The effect of platelet rich plasma combined with microfractures on the treatment of chondral defects: an experimental study in a sheep model. Osteoarthritis and cartilage. 2010 Jul;18(7):971-80.
19. Boffa A, Previtali D, Altamura SA, Zaffagnini S, Candrian C, Filardo G. Platelet-Rich Plasma Augmentation to Microfracture Provides a Limited Benefit for the Treatment of Cartilage Lesions: A Meta-analysis. Orthopaedic journal of sports medicine. 2020 Apr;8(4):2325967120910504.
20. Siclari A, Mascaro G, Gentili C, Kaps C, Cancedda R, Boux E. Cartilage repair in the knee with subchondral drilling augmented with a platelet-rich plasma-immersed polymer-based implant. Knee surgery, sports traumatology, arthroscopy: official journal of the ESSKA. 2014 Jun;22(6):1225-34.
21. Qi YY, Chen X, Jiang YZ, Cai HX, Wang LL, Song XH, et al. Local delivery of autologous platelet in collagen matrix simulated in situ articular cartilage repair. Cell transplantation. 2009;18(10):1161-9.
22. Kreuz PC, Gentili C, Samans B, Martinelli D, Kruger JP, Mittelmeier W, et al. Scaffold-assisted cartilage tissue engineering using infant chondrocytes from human hip cartilage. Osteoarthritis and cartilage. 2013 Dec;21(12):1997-2005.
23. Kon E, Filardo G, Delcogliano M, Fini M, Salamanna F, Giavaresi G, et al. Platelet autologous growth factors decrease the osteochondral regeneration capability of a collagen-hydroxyapatite scaffold in a sheep model. BMC musculoskeletal disorders. 2010 Sep 27;11:220.
24. Perdisa F, Filardo G, Di Matteo B, Marcacci M, Kon E. Platelet rich plasma: a valid augmentation for cartilage scaffolds? A

systematic review. Histology and histopathology. 2014 Jul;29(7):805-14.

25. Dhollander AA, De Neve F, Almqvist KF, Verdonk R, Lambrecht S, Elewaut D, et al. Autologous matrix-induced chondrogenesis combined with platelet-rich plasma gel: technical description and a five pilot patients report. Knee surgery, sports traumatology, arthroscopy : official journal of the ESSKA. 2011 Apr;19(4):536-42.
26. Giannini S, Buda R, Vannini F, Cavallo M, Grigolo B. One-step bone marrow-derived cell transplantation in talar osteochondral lesions. Clinical orthopaedics and related research. 2009 Dec;467(12):3307-20.
27. Buda R, Vannini F, Cavallo M, Baldassarri M, Luciani D, Mazzotti A, et al. One-step arthroscopic technique for the treatment of osteochondral lesions of the knee with bone-marrow-derived cells: three years results. Musculoskeletal surgery. 2013 Aug;97(2):145-51.
28. Giannini S, Buda R, Cavallo M, Ruffilli A, Cenacchi A, Cavallo C, et al. Cartilage repair evolution in post-traumatic osteochondral lesions of the talus: from open field autologous chondrocyte to bone-marrow-derived cells transplantation. Injury. 2010 Nov;41(11):1196-203.
29. Filardo G, Kon E, Roffi A, Di Matteo B, Merli ML, Marcacci M. Platelet-rich plasma: why intra-articular? A systematic review of preclinical studies and clinical evidence on PRP for joint degeneration. Knee surgery, sports traumatology, arthroscopy : official journal of the ESSKA. 2015 Sep;23(9):2459-74.
30. Andriolo L, Di Matteo B, Kon E, Filardo G, Venieri G, Marcacci M. PRP Augmentation for ACL Reconstruction. BioMed research international. 2015;2015:371746.
31. Filardo G, Di Matteo B, Di Martino A, Merli ML, Cenacchi A, Fornasari P, et al. Platelet-Rich Plasma Intra-articular Knee Injections Show No Superiority Versus Viscosupplementation: A Randomized Controlled Trial. The American journal of sports medicine. 2015 Jul;43(7):1575-82.
32. Assirelli E, Filardo G, Mariani E, Kon E, Roffi A, Vaccaro F, et al. Effect of two different preparations of platelet-rich plasma on synoviocytes. Knee surgery, sports traumatology, arthroscopy : official journal of the ESSKA. 2015 Sep;23(9):2690-703.
33. Park SI, Lee HR, Kim S, Ahn MW, Do SH. Time-sequential modulation in expression of growth factors from platelet-rich plasma (PRP) on the chondrocyte cultures. Molecular and cellular biochemistry. 2012 Feb;361(1-2):9-17.
34. Pereira RC, Scaranari M, Benelli R, Strada P, Reis RL, Cancedda R, et al. Dual effect of platelet lysate on human articular cartilage: a maintenance of chondrogenic potential and a transient proinflammatory activity followed by an inflammation resolution. Tissue engineering Part A. 2013 Jun;19(11-12):1476-88.
35. Kon E, Buda R, Filardo G, Di Martino A, Timoncini A, Cenacchi A, et al. Platelet-rich plasma: intra-articular knee in-

jections produced favorable results on degenerative cartilage lesions. Knee surgery, sports traumatology, arthroscopy : official journal of the ESSKA. 2010 Apr;18(4):472-9.

36. Filardo G, Kon E, Buda R, Timoncini A, Di Martino A, Cenacchi A, et al. Platelet-rich plasma intra-articular knee injections for the treatment of degenerative cartilage lesions and osteoarthritis. Knee surgery, sports traumatology, arthroscopy: official journal of the ESSKA. 2011 Apr;19(4):528-35.
37. Di Martino A, Di Matteo B, Papio T, Tentoni F, Selleri F, Cenacchi A, et al. Platelet-Rich Plasma Versus Hyaluronic Acid Injections for the Treatment of Knee Osteoarthritis: Results at 5 Years of a Double-Blind, Randomized Controlled Trial. The American journal of sports medicine. 2019 Feb;47(2):347-54.
38. Previtali D, Merli G, Di Laura Frattura G, Candrian C, Zaffagnini S, Filardo G. The Long-Lasting Effects of "Placebo Injections" in Knee Osteoarthritis: A Meta-Analysis. Cartilage. 2020 Mar 18:1947603520906597.
39. Filardo G, Previtali D, Napoli F, Candrian C, Zaffagnini S, Grassi A. PRP Injections for the Treatment of Knee Osteoarthritis: A Meta-Analysis of Randomized Controlled Trials. Cartilage. 2020 Jun 19:1947603520931170.
40. Altamura SA, Di Martino A, Andriolo L, Boffa A, Zaffagnini S, Cenacchi A, et al. Platelet-Rich Plasma for Sport-Active Patients with Knee Osteoarthritis: Limited Return to Sport. BioMed research international. 2020;2020:8243865.
41. Jevsevar DS. Treatment of osteoarthritis of the knee: evidence-based guideline, 2nd edition. The Journal of the American Academy of Orthopaedic Surgeons. 2013 Sep;21(9):571-6.
42. Bannuru RR, Osani MC, Vaysbrot EE, Arden NK, Bennell K, Bierma-Zeinstra SMA, et al. OARSI guidelines for the non-surgical management of knee, hip, and polyarticular osteoarthritis. Osteoarthritis and cartilage. 2019 Nov;27(11):1578-89.
43. Bruyere O, Honvo G, Veronese N, Arden NK, Branco J, Curtis EM, et al. An updated algorithm recommendation for the management of knee osteoarthritis from the European Society for Clinical and Economic Aspects of Osteoporosis, Osteoarthritis and Musculoskeletal Diseases (ESCEO). Seminars in arthritis and rheumatism. 2019 Dec;49(3):337-50.
44. Arnoczky SP, Sheibani-Rad S. The basic science of platelet-rich plasma (PRP): what clinicians need to know. Sports medicine and arthroscopy review. 2013 Dec;21(4):180-5.

CHAPTER 6

BIOLOGICAL PRODUCTS AND BIOMATERIALS FOR TENDON REGENERATION

Milena Fini, Francesca Veronesi

Complex structure Surgical Sciences and Technologies,
Rizzoli RIT (Research Innovation Technology) Department, IRCCS Rizzoli Orthopaedic Institute

The tendon is characterized by a white and elastic fibrillar structure due to its hypovascular nature [1]. 20% of the total volume of the tendon is occupied by cells, 90-95% of which is represented by tenoblasts and tenocytes that have the function of forming and maintaining the extracellular matrix (ECM) of the tendon [2] (fig. 1).
The ECM of the tendon is composed of 60-80% water, and the remaining 20-40% is represented by Type I Collagen (COLL I), which makes up 95% of collagens, COLL III, V, and XII, which represent 1-5% of collagens, glycosaminoglycans (GAG), glycoproteins and proteoglycans (PG), while elastin accounts for 2% of tendon mass. COLL III plays an important role in the repair process and produces thinner and poorly organized fibrils; COLL V is interspersed with COLL I fibrils and modulates fibril growth, while COLL XII has the ability to bind PG, fibromodulin, and decorin [3] (fig. 2).
Despite what may seem a simple composition, the tendon is a hierarchically very complex structure that is altered

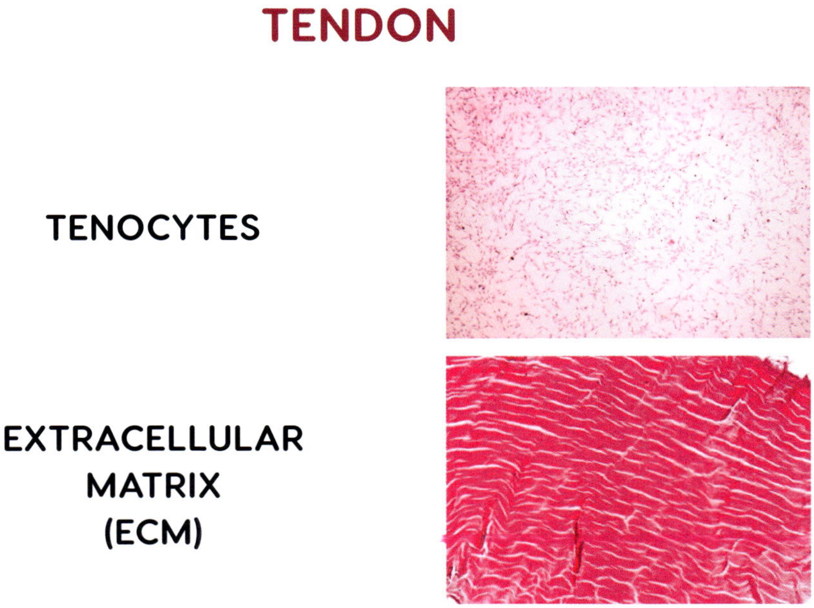

Figure 1 Main components of the tendon: Tenocytes and Extracellular Matrix (ECM)

EXTRACELLULAR MATRIX (ECM)

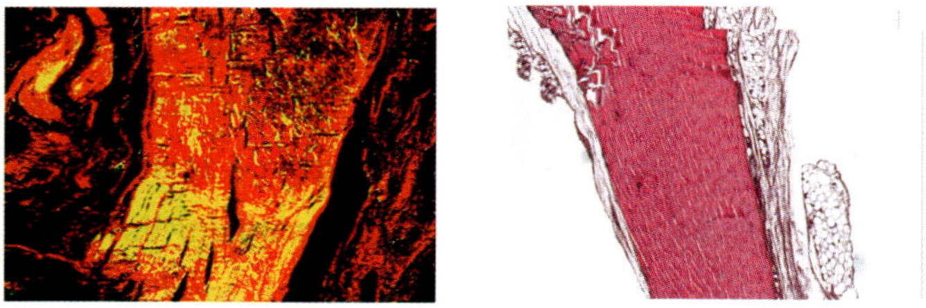

H_2O 60-80%
COLLAGEN I 95% of collagens
COLLAGEN III, IV, V, VI 1-5% of collagens
PROTEOGLYCANS
ELASTIN 2 %

20-40%

Figure 2 Composition of the Extracellular Matrix of the Tendon (ECM)

by different conditions, intrinsic and extrinsic, such as genetic factors, the presence of comorbidities (such as diabetes, hypercholesterolemia, obesity, Cushing's syndrome, and acromegaly), hormonal alterations (deficiency of growth hormone and alterations of thyroid hormones, estrogen, and androgens), aging and physical inactivity.

With aging, COLL content decreases with an increase in markers of senescence, including advanced glycation end (AGE) and senescence-associated beta-gal (SA-β gal), metalloproteinase (MMP), a group of proteolytic enzymes, and degradation products of coll. In addition, there is a reduction in the mechanical strength of the tendon, proliferation, and migration of tenocytes [4].

In addition to aging, estrogen deficiency from the postmenopausal period also plays a fundamental role in the structure of the tendons and the activity of its cells. During the premenopausal period, women show a low risk of tendinopathies, which increases after menopause. Estrogen deficiency reduces COLL turnover, fiber diameter, mechanical properties, and tendon elasticity [5].

An in vitro study evaluated and compared the proliferation and metabolism of tenocytes isolated from Achilles tendons of young, mature, and ovariectomized rats (to simulate postmenopausal estrogen deficiency) in a micro-wound model to simulate and evaluate the tendon regeneration process in vitro. The results highlighted how aging and, more significantly, estrogen deficiency negatively impaired tendon metabolism and regeneration. It was observed that tenocytes taken from mature and ovariectomized rats showed lower cell proliferation, COLL I production, aggress, and elastin than tenocytes taken from young rats. In addition, estrogen deficiency-induced a more significant reduction in fibronectin and elastin and increased MMP than aging. In addition, tenocytes from mature and ovariectomized animals reduced micro-wound regeneration in vitro, with values worse in estrogen deficiency than in aging [5].

As for physical activity, a sedentary lifestyle or sudden interruption of physical activity also compromise the normal structure and properties of the tendon, with alterations in the organization and mechanical properties of the tissue. This underlines that after a period of inactivity (due, for example, to an injury), physical activity should be resumed with caution, following a targeted rehabilitation program [6].

In vivo, this topic was evaluated in trained, untrained rats or 4 weeks after discontinuation of physical activity. The content of PG, COLL I, and fiber organization showed lower values in the patellar tendons of untrained rats or after cessation of physical activity, with increased COLL III, compared to the results of trained rats. Worse results were obtained after the cessation of physical activity, emphasizing that moderate physical activity has a positive effect on the structure of the patellar tendon, while the sudden cessation of physical activity shows a negative effect [7]. It is also reported that the treatment, through repeated injections of hyaluronic acid into the tendon, counteracts tendon degeneration from sudden cessation of physical activity or physical inactivity through an increase in the number of mitochondria and the activity of the wrinkled endoplasmic reticulum, cell proliferation, and viability, COLL I, fibronectin, attack Tenascin-C and a reduction in interleukin 1 β (IL1 β) and MMP13 [8, 9]. In vitro studies have also confirmed that tenocytes, isolated from Achilles tendons of trained subjects, produced more COLL I and PG and less tumor necrosis factor α (TNF α) than tenocytes taken from sedentary subjects [10].

Tendon injuries are classified as chronic degenerative tendinopathies or acute ruptures. Tendinopathy is a continuous and localized pathological event that leads to tissue degeneration, functional weakness, and inflammation and, if stress exceeds the physiological resistance of the tendon, it can also lead to a traumatic rupture [11, 12].

In tendinopathy, the tendon appears thin, irregular, and dark in color with an increased number of tenocytes, irregularly shaped and apoptotic, disorganization of COLL, and neovascularization, with abnormal vessels. Subsequently, in chronic tendinopathy, mucoid or lipoid degeneration, the presence of fibrocartilage or calcium deposits, and increased expression of COLL III is observed [13, 14] (fig. 3). Chronic tendinopathy is one of the primary causes of alterations in locomotion and chronic pain, progressively reducing daily activities and increasing sedentariness, a well-known risk factor for numerous pathologies. However, with chronic tendinopathy typical of old age, current therapies fail. Surgical procedures often cannot be applied in the elderly due to the patient's fragility, and to this, it must be added that the tendon of an elderly person has a poor capacity for regeneration if injured [12].

Among the tendons most affected by tendinopathies, we remember those that make up the rotator cuff and the Achilles tendon.

Rotator cuff lesions are responsible

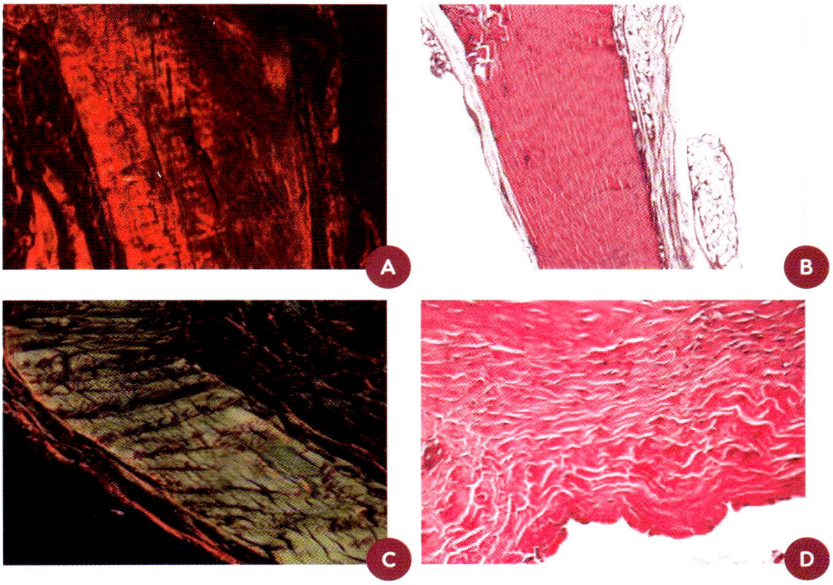

Figure 3 Histological images of healthy (A, B) and tendinopathic (C, D) tendons. Staining Picrosirius Red (A, C), hematoxylin eosin (B, D). The fibers of COLL II are identified in green-yellow and those of COLL I in red-orange (A, C).

for 67% of shoulder pain and reduced function in patients between 40 and 65, with an incidence of 200,000–300,000/year globally and 20-70% of relapses [15].

The Achilles tendon is the most frequently injured (about 40% of all tendon ruptures) in young, middle-aged, or elderly subjects who do recreational activities or unconventional activities. Its incidence increases due to the ever-increasing number of elderly people who dedicate themselves to sports activities. The incidence of relapses after conservative treatments is 12-18%, 1-3% after surgery, with 4-17% of postoperative complications [16].

Spontaneous tendon regeneration is a complex process that usually leads to scar and fibrovascular tissue formation with lower mechanical properties than the original healthy tissue.

Under normal conditions, spontaneous regeneration is slow due to the complex structure of the tendon and its hypocellular and hypovascular nature. Even after one year after the injury, the structure and function of the tissue remain inferior to those of a healthy tendon [17]. The diameter of the collagen fibers is altered, favoring the formation of thinner fibrils with a reduction in the mechanical strength of the tendon. It has also been shown that there is a reduction in regenerative capacity as the size of the lesion increases [18].

For these reasons, the tendon is the tissue of choice for a regenerative therapy approach, with therapeutic strategies that are aimed not at repairing but at regenerating the tissue, through the use mainly of biological treatments: cells, including mainly mesenchymal stem cells (MSCs); growth factors, including platelet-rich plasma (PRP); biomaterials and scaffolds with particular biological and mechanical properties [19].

Among the most used cells for tendon regeneration, we remember the MSCs, thanks to their ability to differentiate, to low immunogenicity, and to trophic effect understood as the ability to produce and release paracrine factors, including growth factors and chemotactic molecules that can recruit other cells at the site of injury. Several sources of MSC have currently been identified, including bone marrow, adipose tissue, periosteum, blood, synovial fluid, muscle, hair follicles, placenta, and dermis. However, the most clinically used sites for tendinopathies of the Achilles tendon, elbow tendons, patella, and rotator cuff are bone marrow, adipose tissue, and placenta [20].

Over the years, we have tried to study, in increasingly advanced in vitro models, the effect of MSCs in tendon regeneration. Although bone marrow MSCs (BMSCs) remain the most widely used, MSCs taken from adipose tissue (ADSCs) show numerous advantages over BMSCs. ADSCs are readily available and isolated from tissue, with minor or absent postoperative complications, high proliferation, and angiogenic capacities, and the influence of aging on viability and differentiation compared to BMSCs [21]. An in vitro study observed a mutual interaction between ADSC and tenocytes. When placed in contact in indirect co-colture with tenocytes, ADSCs increased the viability, gene expression of Decorina and Tenascin, and the rate of migration of tenocytes, while tenocytes increased gene expression ADSC growth factors [22].

In the same indirect co-culture model, but under estrogen deficiency conditions, similar results were obtained. More precisely, the effect of ADSCs under normal conditions and estrogen deficiency was compared, and cell types demonstrated proliferation and migration characteristics, decorin expression, COLL I and Tenascin, and reduced COLL III expression in tenocytes [23].

One of the most widely used biological treatments for tendon regeneration is PRP, a natural concentrate of autologous growth factors that can be injected locally in physiological proportions, minimally invasively, and without adverse effects. The concentration of platelets is about 2-5 times greater than that of peripheral blood. The growth factors that are most commonly contained in the granules α platelets are the platelet-BB-derived growth reflector (PDGF-BB), the transforming growth factor β 1 (TGF-β 1), epidermal growth factors (EGF), insulin growth factor (IGF), vascular endothelial growth factor (VEGF), basic fibroblast growth factor (bFGF) and hepatocyte growth factor (HGF). Preclinical studies, both in vitro and in vivo, have confirmed that PRP promotes tendon neovascularization, cell differentiation, and proliferation, improves mechanical properties, COLL fiber orientation, gene expression, and the production of tendon ECM components, and induces a reduction in pain and inflammation [24].

However, controversial results have been obtained in the clinic due to the heterogeneity of the different formulations of PRP (with a different number of growth factors, cell type, and method of concentration or activation), the nature of the tendinopathies, the treatment protocol (number and timing of injection), and the methods of storage and use (fresh or frozen) [25, 26].

In vitro, the effect of the PRP preservation method and the additive effect of BMSC and PRP on tendon regeneration were evaluated. In this regard, an advanced in vitro model of BMSC-tenocyte and micro-wound co-cultures have been set up. It was observed that BMSCs improved tenocyte migration, micro-wound healing rate, and fibronectin and COLL I production with an additive effect in the presence of PRP. It was also observed that fresh PRP induced significantly better results than frozen PRP in all parameters analyzed [27].

In addition to cells and growth factors, another major actor involved in tissue regenerative medicine is biomaterial (or scaffold), the means by which growth factors, cells, or other biological factors enter the site of injury to improve its regeneration, to give mechanical support to the tissue, to prevent the risk of re-breakage and to allow infiltration, the growth, and differentiation of host tissue cells. The ideal biomaterial should possess rapid degradation to avoid the formation of granulation tissue, a fibrous capsule, or the release of degradation products, induce the release of factors useful for regeneration, be biocompatible, have adequate rigidity, have an easy surgical application, and improve long-term results [28].

Biomaterials can be natural, synthetic, or hybrid. Biomaterials are mostly used in rotator cuff surgery and Achilles tendon surgery in the clinic. The histograms in Fig.4 summarize the synthetic and natural biomaterials most used in the clinic in the last 10 years to regenerate the rotator cuff and Achilles tendon. Natural origin factors are more used than synthetic ones, and among the natural ones, PRP is the most adapted for the regeneration of the rotator cuff, while autologous tissue for the Achilles tendon [29].

In recent years, interest in biomaterials of natural origin for tissue regeneration, such as decellularized ECM matrices, has further increased. Unlike synthetic polymers, such matrices offer temporary mechanical support and a balance of biological and biomechanical stimuli for the regeneration process, thanks to active biological

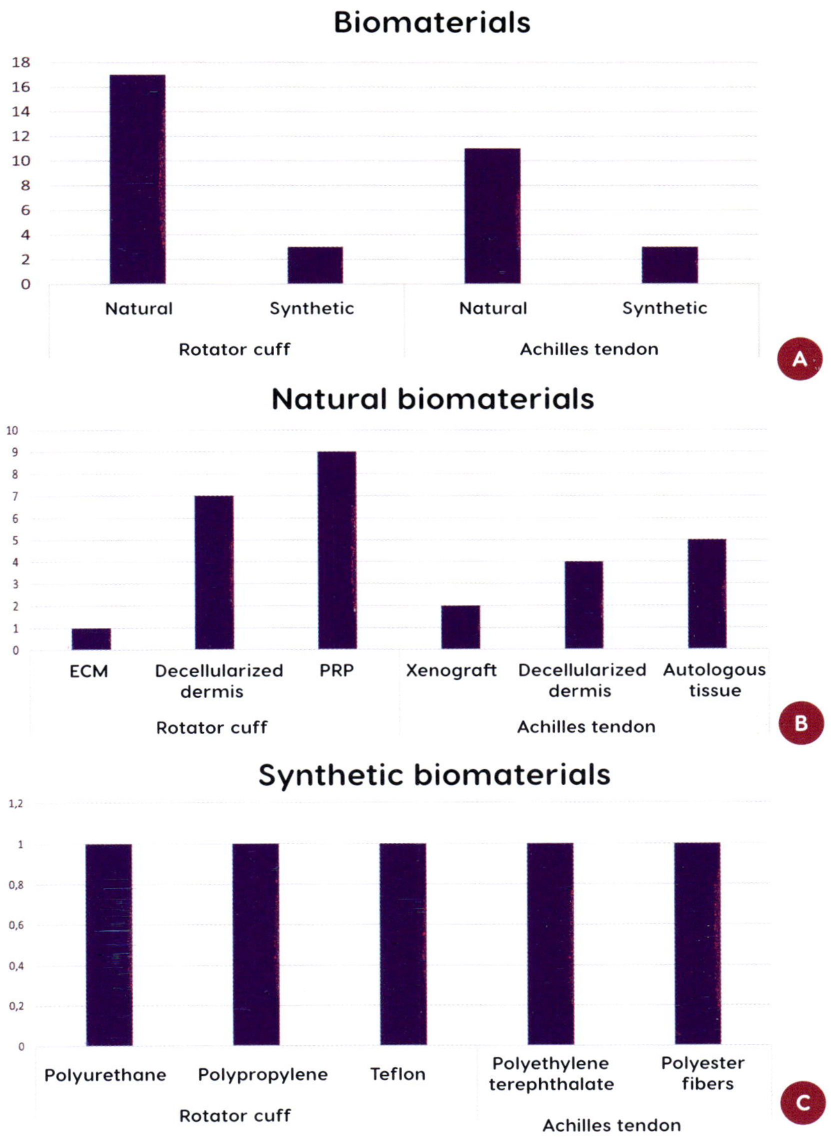

Figure 4 Graphic representation of the quantity and type of biomaterials that have most frequently been used in the clinic for the regeneration of rotator cuff tendons and Achilles tendon in the last 10 years. A) Subdivision into natural and synthetic biomaterials; B) Most widely used natural biomaterials; C) Most widely used synthetic biomaterials.

molecules. In addition, molecules produced after the degradation of these biomaterials play a role in the recruitment and proliferation of cells with a reported antibacterial effect. On the market, there are different types of ECM obtained from dermis, submucosa of the small intestine, pericardium, and fascia lata of different origins, human, swine, bovine or equine. The CME of human origin is classified as a transplant, and each country follows specific rules for controlling human-derived tissues. Recently in Italy, the Large Burns Center of Cesena, in collaboration with the Rizzoli Orthopedic Institute, has patented chemical-physical decellularization of the allogeneic human dermis taken from multi-organ and multi woven donors. To evaluate the absence of viable cells and, at the same time, the maintenance of the matrix structure, biological, histological, and ultrastructural analyzes were carried out demonstrating the effectiveness of decellularization and the maintenance of the matrix in terms of biomechanical and bioactivity. Good mechanical properties of the decellularized dermis have been demonstrated without the onset of inflammatory reactions [30]. In vitro tenocytes seeded on the decellularized dermis increased the production of COLL I, fibronectin, PG, and TGF β 1 and dermis extracts, improved the regeneration time of a micro-wound set up in vitro [31].

In the clinic, the decellularized dermis was used as augmentation in 5 patients suffering from massive rotator cuff lesions and degeneration of the supraspinate and infraspinate tendons. After 1 year from surgery, 3 patients demonstrate a complete regeneration, 1 patient a partial re-rupture, and 1 re-rupture. In addition, the absence of adverse inflammatory reactions or septic complications was observed, laying the foundation for a prospective controlled study [32].

Biomaterials and scaffolds can be used as a vehicle for cells and growth factors and promote the regenerative process of tissue and prevent the formation of peritendinous adhesions after tendon surgery. They can act as a barrier to block the infiltration of fibroblasts without interfering with the passage of cytokines and growth factors into the surgical site of regeneration.

An in vivo study performed an acute Achilles tendon injury model bilaterally in rats. This lesion was sutured with Kessler's technique, and a biomaterial based on COLL I was applied around the surgical site. After 8 and 16 weeks, a reduction in peritendinous adhesions and the formation of COLL III was observed. On the other hand, there was an improvement in the production of COLL I and the elastic modulus [33].

Conclusions

Translational research with the collaboration of researchers and clinicians has led to numerous innovations in regenerative and reparative tendon medicine. To carefully evaluate the impact of new technologies, it is necessary to set up reliable and advanced experimental models starting from the clinical needs in terms of safety, sustainability, and feasibility of the numerous therapies that can currently be developed.

References

1. Li HY, Hua YH. Achilles tendinopathy: current concepts about the basic science and clinical treatments. Biomed Res Int 2016;2016:6492597.
2. Roche AJ, Calder JDF. Achilles tendinopathy: a review of the current concepts of treatment. Bone Joint J 2013;95:1299-1307.
3. Ribbans WJ, Collins M. Pathology of the tendo Achillis: do our genes contribute? J Bone Joint Surg 2013;95:305-313.
4. Lui PPY, Wong CM. Biology of Tendon Stem Cells and Tendon in Aging. Front Genet 2020;10:1338.
5. Torricelli P, Veronesi F, Pagani S, Maffulli N, Masiero S, Frizziero A, Fini M. In vitro tenocyte metabolism in aging and oestrogen deficiency. Age (Dordr) 2013;35:2125-2136.
6. Frizziero A, Salamanna F, Della Bella E, Vittadini F, Gasparre G, Nicoli Aldini N, Masiero S, Fini M. The Role of Detraining in Tendon Mechanobiology. Front Aging Neurosci 2016;8:43.
7. Frizziero A, Fini M, Salamanna F, Veicsteinas A, Maffulli N, Marini M. Effect of training and sudden detraining on the patellar tendon and its enthesis in rats. BMC Musculoskelet Disord 2011;12:20.
8. Frizziero A, Salamanna F, Giavaresi G, Ferrari A, Martini L, Marini M, Veicstei-

nas A, Maffulli N, Masiero S, Fini M. Hyaluronic acid injections protect patellar tendon from detraining-associated damage. Histol Histopathol 2015;30:1079-1088.

9. Salamanna F, Frizziero A, Pagani S, Giavaresi G, Curzi D, Falcieri E, Marini M, Abruzzo PM, Martini L, Fini M. Metabolic and cytoprotective effects of in vivo peri-patellar hyaluronic acid injections in cultured tenocytes. Connect Tissue Res 2015;56:35-43.
10. Franchi M, Torricelli P, Giavaresi G, Fini M. Role of moderate exercising on Achilles tendon collagen crimping patterns and proteoglycans. Connect Tissue Res 2013;54:267-74.
11. Steven BW. Achilles tendon disorders. Med Clin N Am 2014;98:331-338.
12. Nourissat G, Houard X, Sellam J, Duprez D, Berenbaum F. Use of autologous growth factors in aging tendon and chronic tendinopathy. Front Biosci (Elite Ed) 2013;5:911-921.
13. Kirchgesner T, Larbi A, Omoumi P, et al. Drug-induced tendinopathy: from physiology to clinical applications. Joint Bone Spine 2014;81:485-492.
14. Knobloch K. The role of tendon microcirculation in Achilles and patellar tendinopathy. J Orthop Surg Res 2008;3:18.
15. Mahon HS, Christensen JE, Brockmeier SF. Shoulder Rotator Cuff Pathology: Common Problems and Solutions. Clin Sports Med 2018;37:179-196.
16. Wegrzyn J, Luciani JF, Philippot R, Brunet-Guedj E, Moyen B, Besse JL. Chronic Achillies tendon rupture reconstruction using a modified flexor hallucis longus transfer. Int Orthop 2010;34:1187–1192.
17. Liu CF, Aschbacher-Smith L, Barthelery NJ, et al. What we should know before using tissue egineering techniques to repair injured tendons: a developmental biology perspective. Tissue Eng Part B-Rev 2011;17:165–176.
18. Matthews TJ, Hand GC, Rees JL, et al. Pathology of the torn rotator cuff tendon. Reduction in potential for repair as tear size increases. J Bone Joint Surg Br 2006;88:489-495.
19. Lipman K, Wang C, Ting K, Soo C, Zheng Z. Tendinopathy: injury, repair, and current exploration. Drug Des Devel Ther 2018;12:591-603.
20. Veronesi F, Salamanna F, Tschon M, Maglio M, Nicoli Aldini N, Fini M. Mesenchymal stem cells for tendon healing: what is on the horizon? J Tissue Eng Regen Med 2017;11:3202-3219.
21. Veronesi F, Pagani S, Della Bella E, Giavaresi G, Fini M. Estrogen deficiency does not decrease the in vitro osteogenic potential of rat adipose-derived mesenchymal stem cells. Age (Dordr) 2014;36:9647.
22. Veronesi F, Torricelli P, Della Bella E, Pagani S, Fini M. In vitro mutual interaction between tenocytes and adipose-derived mesenchymal stromal cells. Cytotherapy 2015;17:215-223.
23. Veronesi F, Della Bella E, Torricelli P, Pa-

gani S, Fini M. Effect of adipose-derived mesenchymal stromal cells on tendon healing in aging and estrogen deficiency: an in vitro co-culture model. Cytotherapy 2015;17:1536-1544.

24. Salamanna F, Veronesi F, Maglio M, Della Bella E, Sartori M, Fini M. New and emerging strategies in platelet-rich plasma application in musculoskeletal regenerative procedures: general overview on still open questions and outlook. Biomed Res Int 2015;2015:846045.
25. Filardo G, Di Matteo B, Kon E, Merli G, Marcacci M. Platelet-rich plasma in tendon-related disorders: results and indications. Knee Surg Sports Traumatol Arthrosc 2018;26:1984-1999.
26. Andia I, Maffulli N. Muscle and tendon injuries: the role of biological interventions to promote and assist healing and recovery. Arthroscopy 2015;31:999-1015.
27. Veronesi F, Pagani S, Torricelli P, Filardo G, Cavallo C, Grigolo B, Fini M. PRP and MSCs on tenocytes artificial wound healing: an in vitro study comparing fresh and frozen PRP. Histol Histopathol 2018;33:1323-1334.
28. Ratcliffe A, Butler DL, Dyment NA, Cagle PJJr, Proctor CS, Ratcliffe SS, Flatow EL. Scaffolds for tendon and ligament repair and regeneration. Annals Biomed Eng 2015;43:819–831.
29. Veronesi F, Borsari V, Contartese D, Xian J, Baldini N, Fini M. The clinical strategies for tendon repair with biomaterials: A review on rotator cuff and Achilles tendons. J Biomed Mater Res B Appl Biomater 2020;108:1826-1843.
30. Bondioli E, Fini M, Veronesi F, Giavaresi G, Tschon M, Cenacchi G, Cerasoli S, Giardino R, Melandri D. Development and evaluation of a decellularized membrane from human dermis. J Tissue Eng Regen Med 2014;8:325-336.
31. Fini M, Bondioli E, Castagna A, Torricelli P, Giavaresi G, Rotini R, Marinelli A, Guerra E, Orlandi C, Carboni A, Aiti A, Benedettini E, Giardino R, Melandri D. Decellularized human dermis to treat massive rotator cuff tears: in vitro evaluations. Connect Tissue Res 2012;53:298-306.
32. Rotini R, Marinelli A, Guerra E, Bettelli G, Castagna A, Fini M, Bondioli E, Busacca M. Human dermal matrix scaffold augmentation for large and massive rotator cuff repairs: preliminary clinical and MRI results at 1-year follow-up. Musculoskelet Surg 2011;95 Suppl 1:S13-23.
33. Veronesi F, Giavaresi G, Bellini D, Casagranda V, Pressato D, Fini M. Evaluation of a new collagen-based medical device (ElastiCo®) for the treatment of acute Achilles tendon injury and prevention of peritendinous adhesions: An in vitro biocompatibility and in vivo investigation. J Tissue Eng Regen Med 2020;14:1113-1125.

CHAPTER 7

REGENERATIVE THERAPY IN OSTEOARTHRITIS

Sandro Giannini[1], Antonio Mazzotti[2]

1) Professor Emeritus, IRCCS Rizzoli Orthopaedic Institute, University of Bologna, Italy

2) 1st Orthopaedic and Traumatologic Clinic, IRCCS Istituto Ortopedico Rizzoli, Department of Biomedical and Neuromotor Sciences, University of Bologna, Italy

Introduction

In degenerative arthritic forms, the goal of treatment has always been to resolve the painful symp-toms and, at the same time to maintain a certain functionality during ordinary daily activities.

The initial treatment uses medical, orthotic, and rehabilitative conservative measures. For cases that are poorly responsive to conservative treatment, surgical treatment may emerge, which provides dif-ferent options, depending on the patient's pathological anatomy and characteristics. Traditionally, treatment options include joint fusion (arthrodesis) or prosthetic replacement, with different func-tional results depending on the anatomical district concerned.

The evolution of surgical techniques in the treatment of arthritic lesions, together with the most re-cent research achievements, has led to the development of methods that are increasingly attentive to biology and based on tissue regeneration, especially in young and active patients.

Over the years, numerous biological treatments for cartilage lesions [1-4] have been proposed, but only a few of these have demonstrated the ability to reconstruct damaged cartilage [5,6]. In addition, indications for these types of treatments have always been reserved for small osteochondral lesions. In the literature, bone marrow stimulation techniques (drilling, microfractures), transplantation of os-teochondral segments (mosaicplasty), and regenerative techniques (transplantation of autologous chondrocytes, transplantation of mesenchymal stem cells) have been described.

Most of these methods have been shown to achieve good clinical results. However, certain aspects still limit their use: some are able to repair the lesion with only fibrocartilaginous tissue, while others require open surgery and are technically complex.

To overcome these problems, attention has been focused for years on mesenchymal stem cells, able to direct themselves towards a cartilaginous and bone type line and replicate spontaneously, without requiring an

expansion phase in the laboratory [7]. The mesenchymal stem cells, easily taken from the patient's iliac crest, can be implanted after a short process of concentration and elimination of red blood cells that takes place directly in the operating room. This allows to implant in the site of in-jury, in a single surgical intervention, the mesenchymal stem cells, the mononuclear cells, and all those factors present in the bone marrow that constitute a microenvironment with very high regen-erative potential.
Several studies [8-10] have shown a good regeneration of bone and cartilage tissue, with almost complete resolution of the chondral defect and good integration of the regenerated in the medium term in more than 90% of cases.
Given the promising results obtained, these regenerative techniques have recently been applied to pre-arthritic and arthrosis forms in young patients [11,12] in an attempt to avoid or at least delay a prosthetic replacement intervention, which for years has represented the only possible solution.
When performing cartilage repairs, it is important to consider any axial defects of the limb, which must be treated previously or simultaneously by realignment procedures such as corrective osteoto-mies or joint reconstructions.

Regenerative therapy in ankle osteoarthritis

One of the main problems in the treatment of arthritic lesions is the difficulty of reconstructing a native joint surface. This difficulty is all the greater, the more extensive the cartilage lesion. One of the most used classifications for ankle osteoarthritis was proposed by Van Dijk [13] and provided for 4 degrees:

- Grade 0. The joint appears normal or affected solely by subchondral sclerosis.
- Grade 1. Osteophytes are present without narrowing of the articular rhyme.
- Grade 2. There is a narrowing of the rhyme with or without osteophytes.
- Grade 4. Disappearance or total or subtotal deformation of the articular rhyme.

In relation to this classification, you can set a treatment algorithm.
In injuries arthritic lesions up to grade 2, it is possible to perform regenerative treatments in the absence of misalignments.
In grade 2/3 lesions, it is possible to associate regenerative treatments with an arthrodiatasis procedure in the absence of misalignments.
In grade 2/3 lesions, in the presence of misalignments, it is appropriate to resolve the defect on the frontal plane by osteotomies or joint reconstructions in relation to the pathological anatomy.
In grade 3 lesions, as an alternative to traditional treatments of arthrodesis or prosthetic replacement, partial or total osteochondral transplants can be performed in relation to the pathological anatomy.

Arthritic lesions up to grade 2, in the absence of misalignments

After the brilliant results obtained with autologous chondrocyte transplants (fig. 1), the evolutions in tissue engineering techniques have allowed in recent years to apply regenerative techniques through stem cell transplantation and the treatment of pre-arthrosis arthritic ankle lesions, generally up to grade 2 according to VanDijk.
Stem cells give rise to progenitor cells and are distinguished from them by their ability to renew and reproduce by the process of asymmetric cell division. A peculiar characteristic of stem cells is multipotentiality, that is, the ability to differentiate into virtually any other type of tissue: stem cells derived from bone, bone marrow, muscle, and fat, have been shown to be able to differentiate into multiple phenotypes, including bone, cartilage, tendon, ligamentous, adipose, muscular and nervous tissue [14,15]. Sources of stem cells for musculoskeletal tissue are diverse and include bone marrow, cartilage, muscle, and fat. The possibility of withdrawal from these tissues is influenced by the complications that the maneuver inevitably entails. In particular, bone marrow aspiration is more practical, associated with less

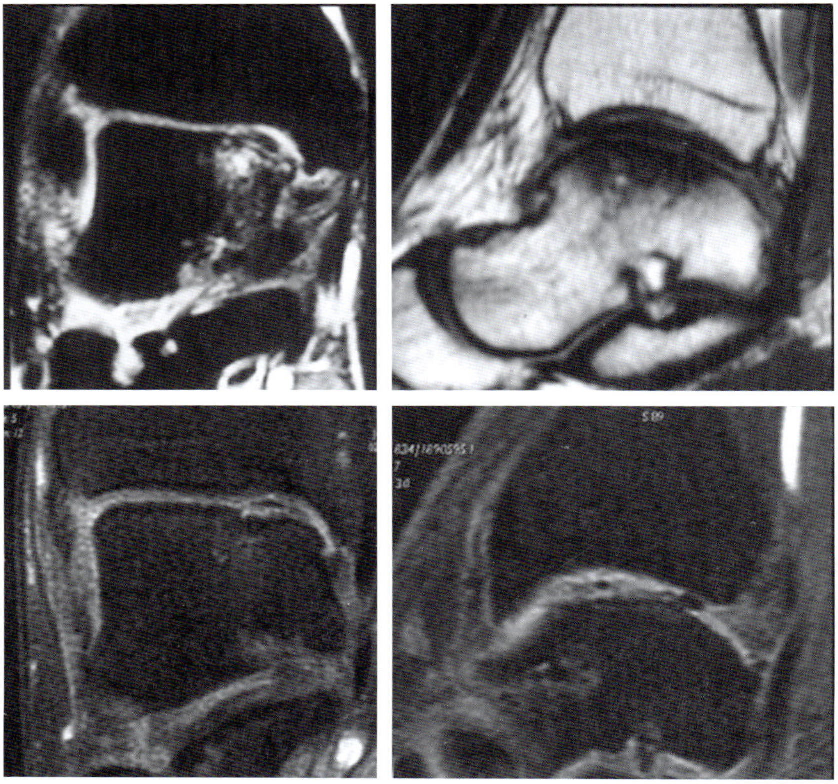

Figure 1 Top: Pre-operative MRI in a 36-year-old male patient with an extensive medial osteochondral lesion at the level of the astragal trochlea. Below MRI 6 months after the transplantation of autologous chondrocytes shows a good regenerated. The implantation of autologous chondrocytes is a procedure in which chondrocytes are collected during a first surgical phase and, subsequently in the laboratory, expanded in culture, sown on unique scaffolds, and then reimplanted during a second surgical inter-vention. Chondrocytes can be taken from the knee, ankle, or, if possible, from a detached osteochon-dral fragment.

morbidity, and allows to obtain a cellular suspension that can be quickly processed, even intra-operatively, for immediate reimplantation.

Mesenchymal stem cells are often used as a pure cell line, i.e., selected after appropriate steps in culture by eliminating cells that do not express the membrane markers typical of mesenchymal stem cells themselves.

Currently, the ability of stem cells to interact biochemically and mechanically with the "surrounding microenvironment" is known, which seems to be able to influence their gene expression and, therefore, the properties of the cells themselves.

This microenvironment is interpreted broadly and includes factors such as the extracellular matrix, the adhesion molecules that mediate cell-to-cell and cell-to-cell contact, numerous growth factors, cytokines, and soluble chemokines.

This aspect supports the choice to use in orthopedic clinical practice, the set of all bone marrow cells, in order to maintain as much as possible the system of mutual interactions active in the bone marrow niche and to transfer to the site of injury the entire regenerative potential present in the mononuclear cellular component of the bone marrow [16].

The use of supports for cell development such as scaffolds has allowed modern bioengineering to propose numerous devices capable of accommodating the implantation and growth of stem cells. The components mainly used in developing such devices are collagen and esterified hyaluronic acid: the degradation of these components does not favor the development of cytotoxic substances. In the particular environment, it can perform positive effects for the growth and engraftment of the transplanted cellular component [17].

The "One-Step" technique presented in 2009 [18] with the subsequent development of the IORG1 device (Novagenit) [9] uses a bone marrow cell concentrate on scaffolds to regenerate cartilage lesions (fig. 2).

The technique involves a first preoperative phase in which peripheral blood is taken to obtain the production of platelet gel used during the intervention.

The surgical phase begins with removing the bone marrow aspirate from the posterosuperior iliac crest to a supine patient, already under anesthesia. The sampling involves the aspiration of 60 ccs of bone marrow blood. The IORG1 System (Novagenit) allows the

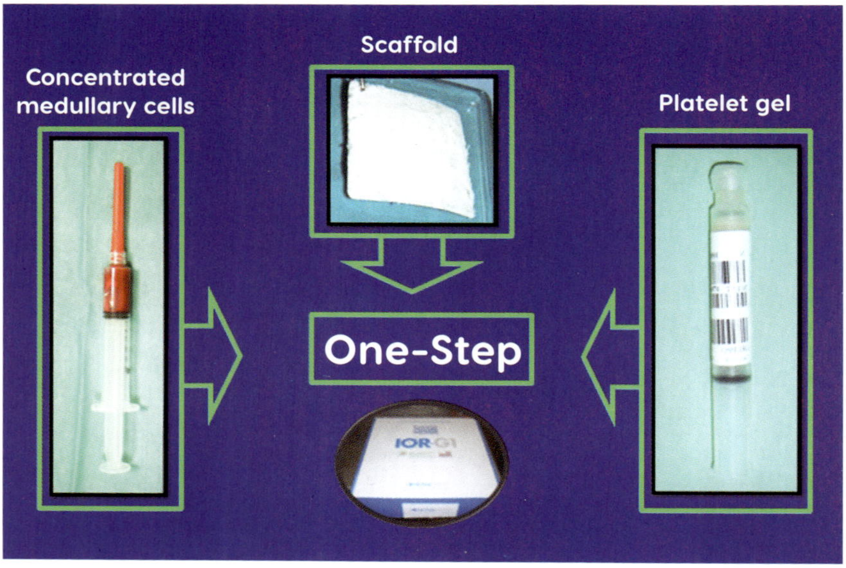

Figure 2 The "One-Step" technique and its components: concentrated medullary cells, scaffolds, platelet gel.

closed-loop preparation of the bone marrow concentrate, reducing the risk of contamination. The concentration mechanism includes a mechanical concentration in the centrifuge and a magnetic one. Both steps take place in the operating room, during the preparation of the sterile ankle field, at the end of which a bone marrow concentrate equal to 6 ccs is obtained.

In most cases, implantation can occur with the arthroscopic method, or, especially in more extensive pre-arthritic or arthrosis lesions, arthroscopically (fig. 3).

The scaffold, collagen, or hyaluronic acid membrane, is sized to the same extent as the lesion and soaked with the previously prepared autologous bone marrow concentrate.

The soaked scaffold is then implanted: the membrane is placed in the lesion bed using a flat spatula until it is perfectly filled.

The previously prepared platelet gel can therefore be applied, with a fun-

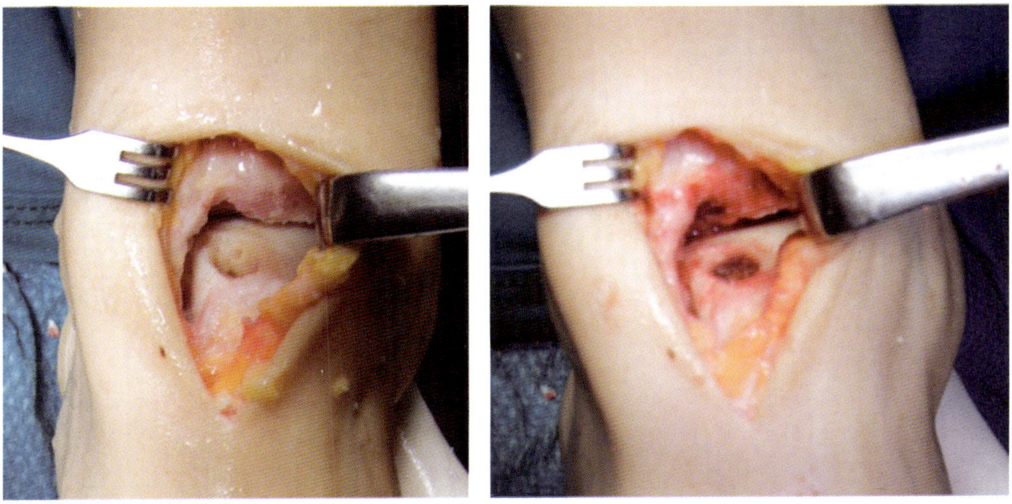

Figure 3 Arthrotomic repair of extensive medial osteochondral lesion at the level of the astragal trochlea

ction and biological, of secondary stabilization of the graft.

The postoperative protocol provides for the early mobilization of the operated ankle: starting from the first postoperative day, the patient performs active and passive movements in flexion extension. Walking is granted with the help of two antibrachials without load on the operated limb for the first 6/7 weeks; a gradual partial load is then granted, with freeloading at 10-12 weeks. Low-impact sports activity (swimming, cycling) is granted 4 months after surgery, while high-impact activities (running, football, tennis, etc ...) are allowed at 10-12 months [16].

The results reported in the literature [10,12,19,20] have shown that the use of mesenchymal cells of bone marrow origin can be a valid option not only for the treatment of osteochondral lesions but also for pre-arthritic and arthritic conditions (figg. 4,5,6), to delay or in some cases avoid more invasive interventions such as prosthetic replacement or arthrodesis.

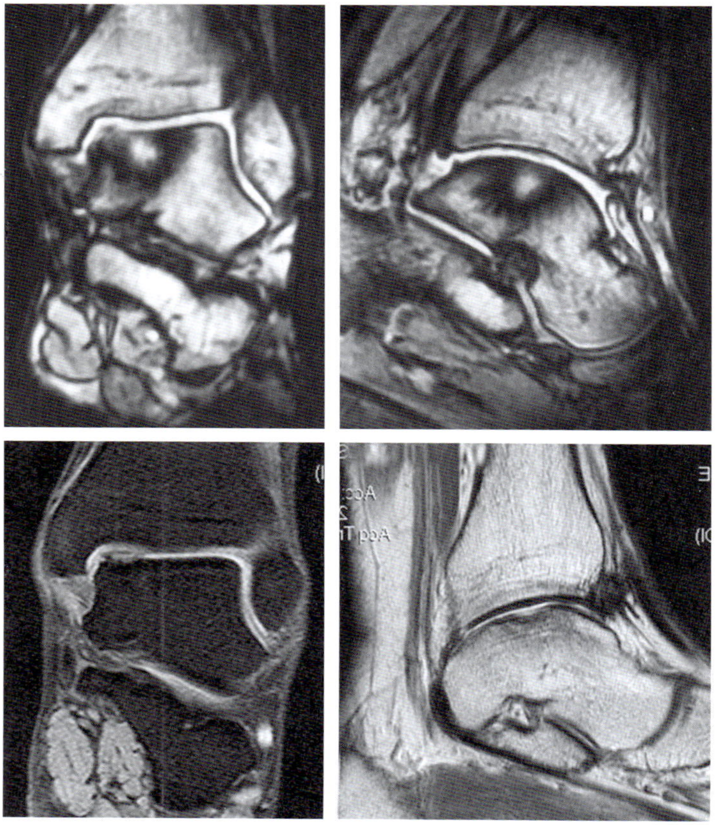

Figure 4 Top: Pre-operative MRI in male patient 32 years. Below MRI 36 months after regenerative treatment with "One-Step" technique

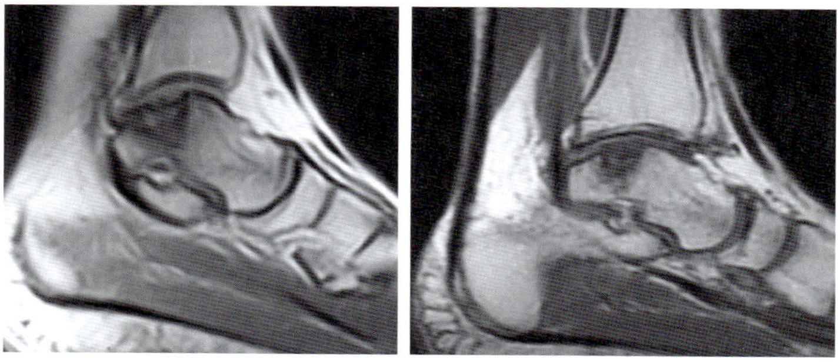

Figure 5 Left: Pre-operative MRI in a 39-year-old female patient. Right MRI 24 months after regenerative treatment with "One-Step" technique

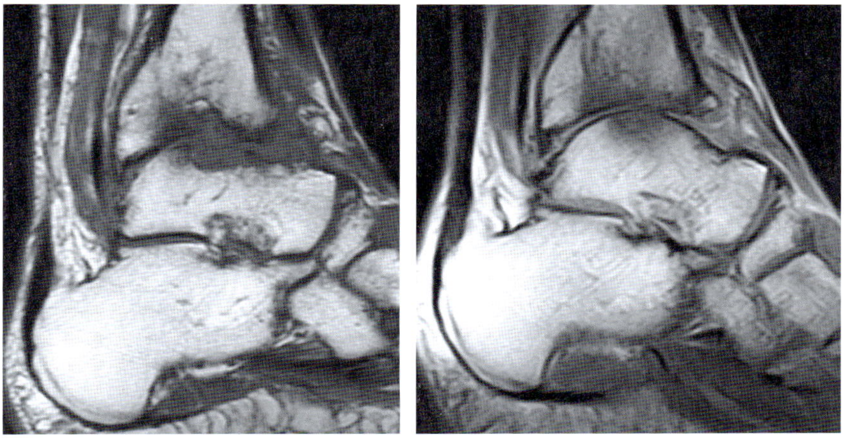

Figure 6 Left: Pre-operative MRI in a 33-year-old male patient, in bimalleolar fracture outcomes with extensive osteochondral lesion. Right MRI 24 months after regenerative treatment with "One-Step" technique

Grade 2/3 lesions, in the absence of misalignments

In grade 2/3 lesions, according to Van-Dijk, in the absence of misalignments, it is possible to associate the regenerative treatment of cartilage with an arthrodiatasis procedure. Arthrodiatasis involves performing a temporary joint distraction using an external fixator, theoretically allows the formation of a fibro-cartilaginous panniculus that can facilitate the sliding of the articular heads and reduce pain at the load.

The surgical technique involves using a monoaxial external fixation system [21] connected to clamps applied medially on the leg, a bridge of the tibiotarsal joint. Usually, two "chips" are applied to the medial surface of the tibia with proximal grip, an astragal "fiche" and a calcaneal one for the distal socket (fig. 7).

The distraction of the apparatus is then performed, constantly verifying the maintenance of the movement of the articulated clamp and the co-axiality between the axis of the external fixator and the tibial axis. It is advisable

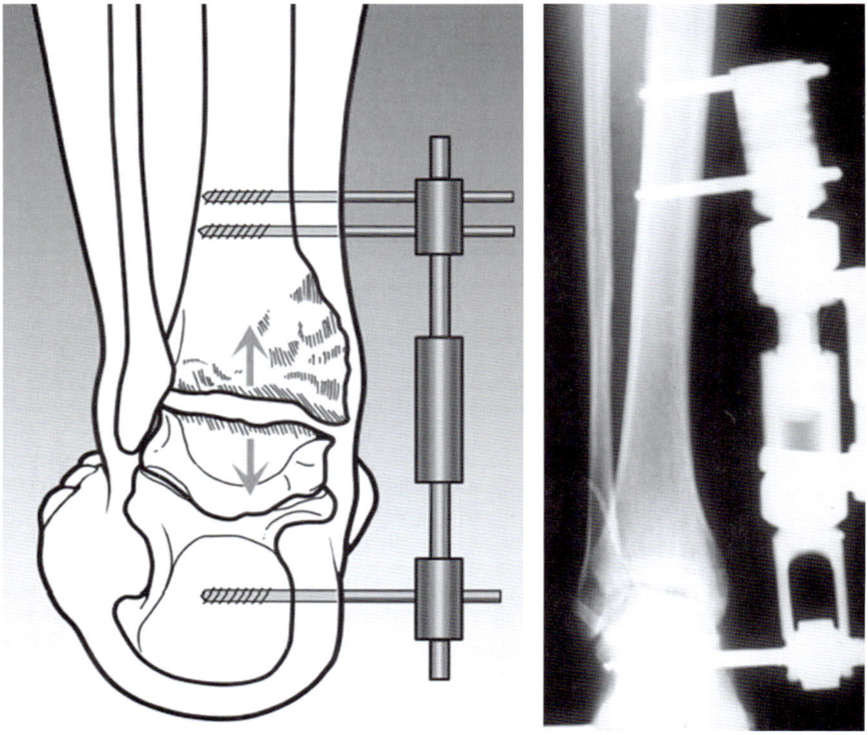

Figure 7 Arthrodiatasis with distraction of the tibio-tarsal joint by mono-axial fixation system

not to exceed a joint diastasis of 4-5 mm, to avoid the risk of complications, such as an algodystrophic syndrome. Distraction can be achieved in a single time or progressively (0.5 mm x 2/ day for the 5 days following surgery) according to the degree of initial joint stiffness [22].

The post-operative protocol provides immediate joint mobilization, possibly performed in analgesia in the first 7-10 days with peridural catheter permanence and infusion with local anesthetics, followed by an early and progressive granting of the load on the operated limb. The implant is removed after 2-3 months, depending on the extent of the joint damage detected, the tolerability of the implant, or any complications.

The long-term results of the experiences with joint distraction performed with an external axial fixator at the level of the tibiotarsal (fig. 8) seem to confirm its initial indication or an alternative method to demolition or more invasive interventions such as arthrodesis or prosthesis.

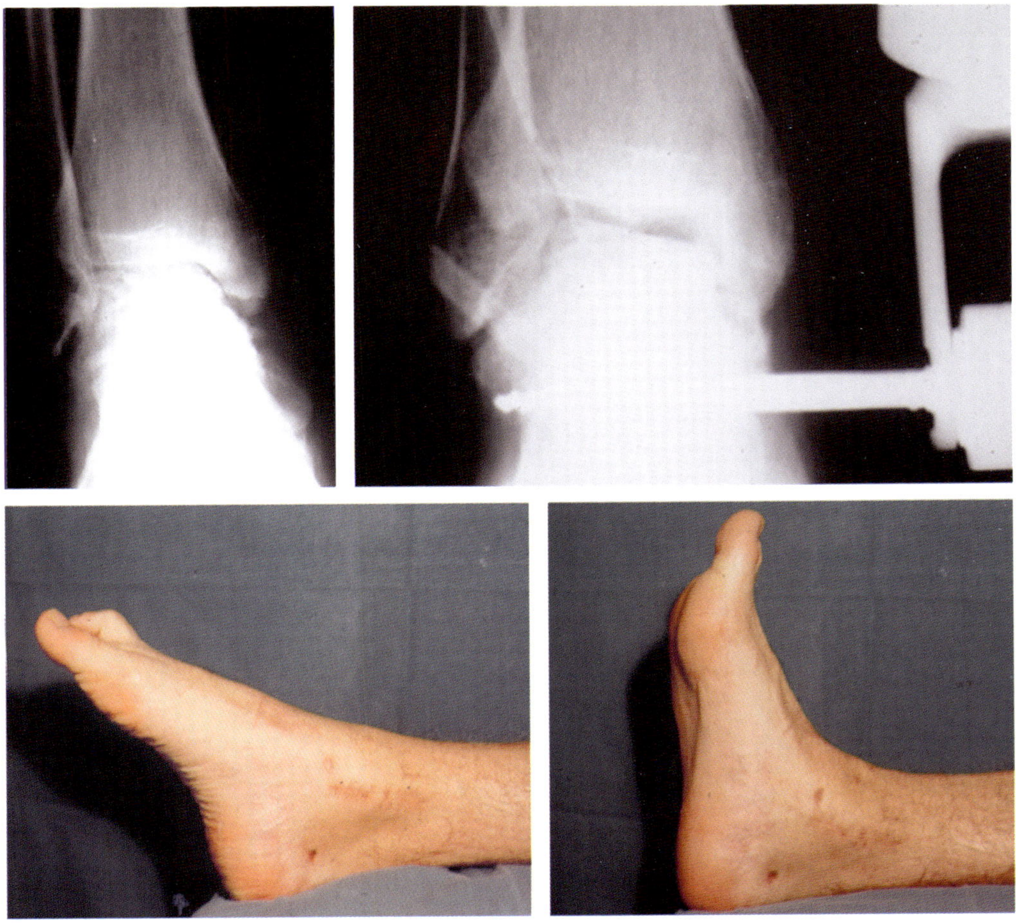

Figure 8 Top left: RX of the ankle in anteroposterior projection, of male patient, 40 years old, showing picture of arthritic degeneration. Top right: RX with joint distraction by means of mono-axial external fixator. At the bottom normo-permitted flexo-extension movements 10 years after treatment

Grade 2/3 lesions, in the presence of misalignments

In grade 2/3 lesions, in the presence of misalignments, in addition to the repair of arthritic damage, it is appropriate to resolve the defect on the frontal axis by osteotomy or joint reconstructions in relation to pathological anatomy [23].
In order to identify any ankle deformities and set up a correct treatment, it is essential to consider some radiographic parameters.
At the tibial level, an anatomical axis is recognized, consisting of the line underlying the indentation between the 2 tibial spines proximal and the center of the conjugation cartilage of the distally tibial plafond. In a tibia with normal anatomy, this axis coincides with the mechanical axis and has a slight variant (1°-2°) with respect to the perpendicular to the ground. Another important axis to evaluate tibial deformities is passing through the tibial articular surface, which intersects the mechanical axis of the tibia in the center of the plafond forming on the frontal plane. The angle was known in the literature as TAS (Tibial-Ankle Surface), open medially, whose normal value in the Caucasian population varies from 91° to 93°. This value describes the slight physiological valgus of the ankle. On the sagittal plane, these same lines form the TLS (Tibial Lateral Surface) angle, opened anteriorly, with normal values between 81° and 82°. In the presence of a deformity, it is important to consider an additional parameter, defined as CORA (Center Of Rotation and Angulation); this is defined as the crossing point between the proximal and distal mechanical axis of the tibia; the angle between them represents the extent of the deformity to be corrected.
Malalignments can be distinguished into supra-articular and articular. In the case of supra-articular malalignments, corrective osteotomies are necessary, while in common defects, reconstructions of the joint must be performed.
Possible corrective osteotomies include:

- Osteotomies in plus (fig. 9): depending on the type of deformity they can be carried out at the level of the

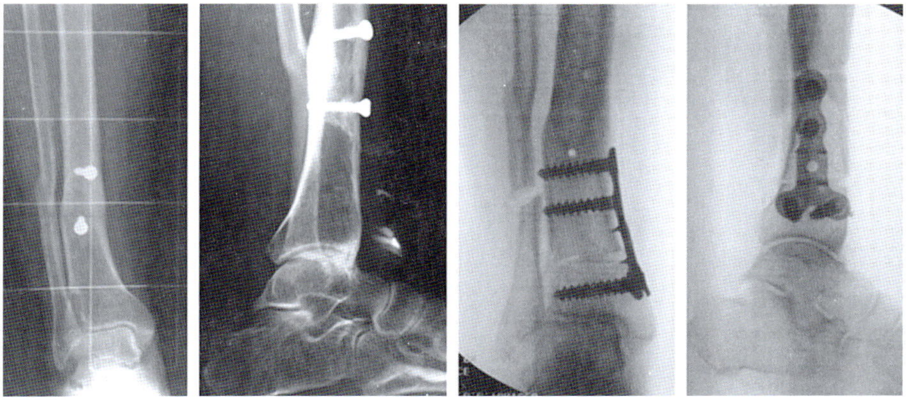

Figure 9 22-year-old male patient, with supra-articular deformity in varus, secondary to malunion of the tibia. Resumption of the chondral lesion is performed in arthroscopy, osteotomy of the fibula and tibial osteotomy in plus with bank bone graft synthesized with plaque

medial or lateral surface of the tibia. They allow the maintenance, or slight increase, of the length of the operated limb. Normally an autologous tricortical bone graft taken from the homolateral iliac crest or an allograft is used. These osteotomies allow multiplex corrections based on the angle of the cut. Compared to osteotomies in minus sometimes require a longer consolidation time

- Osteotomies in minus: they can be performed at the level of the medial or lateral surface of the tibia. Their main disadvantage is the shortening of the operated limb, a factor that must always be considered during pre-operative planning. The absence of grafts and the shorter healing time are the main advantages.
- Peroneal osteotomies: peroneal osteotomies in shortening or elongation are usually indicated in consolidation defects secondary to fractures in the external rotation that cause a shortening with rotation of the fibula. Correction of the deformity of the fibula allows the restoration of joint relationships at the level of the tibio-peroneal syndesmosis.

In case of joint malalignments and cartilage repair, reconstructions of the joint must be performed. These techniques usually involve a reconstruction of the fibula to act on the tibio-peroneal syndesmosis, associating when necessary a ligamentous plastic (figg. 10,11). It is also necessary to correct at the same time any malunion of the posterior malleolus or sinkings of the medial tibial plafond. In other cases, it is possible, once the joint reconstruction has been performed, to practice an arthrodiatasis with an external fixator in distraction (fig. 12)

Grade 3 injuries

Severe osteoarthritis in the young and active patient is a therapeutic problem that is difficult to solve. The arthrodesis of tibiotarsal (fig. 13) has represented for years the only treatment able to solve the advanced degenerative forms. The severe instabilities of this joint are still current practice and in many respects of the first choice. Although reliable and reproducible, with positi-

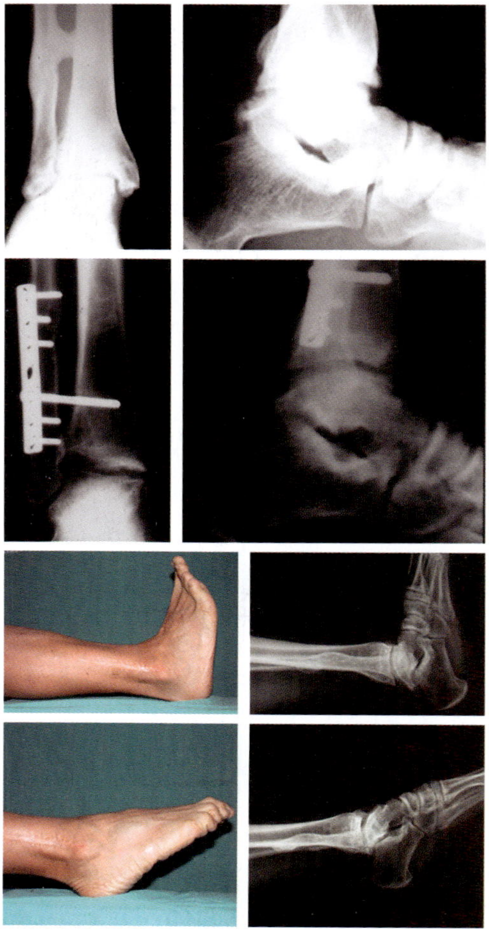

Figure 10 41-year-old male patient. Outcomes of conservatively treated peroneal fracture. At the top, pre-operative X-rays under load show, in anteroposterior, a malunion of the fibula and a post-traumatic tibio-peroneal synostosis. The patient undergoes chondral repair and joint reconstruction with fibula lengthening. At the bottom you can see the good articulation of the ankle at a distance of 8 years from the treatment

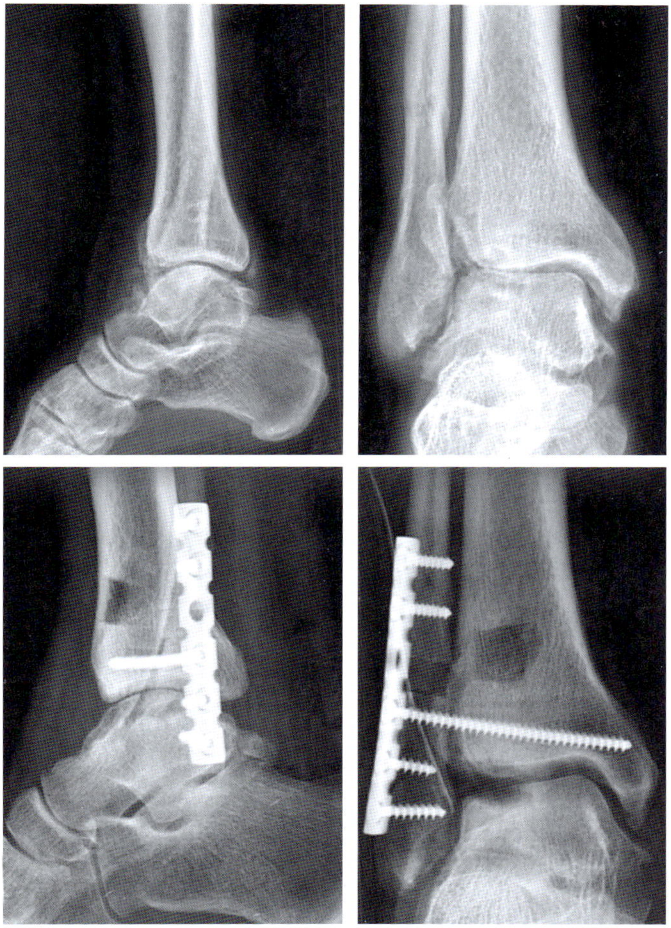

Figure 11 35-year-old female patient. Outcomes of conservatively treated peroneal fracture. At the top, pre-operative X-rays under load show, in anteroposterior, a tibial hyperpressure at the level of the astragal trochlea, a cause of osteochondral injury. The patient undergoes chondral repair surgery by reclamation and implantation of scaffolds with concentrate of autologous bone marrow mononuclear cells and joint reconstruction with elongation of the fibula, (RX below, control at 12 months).

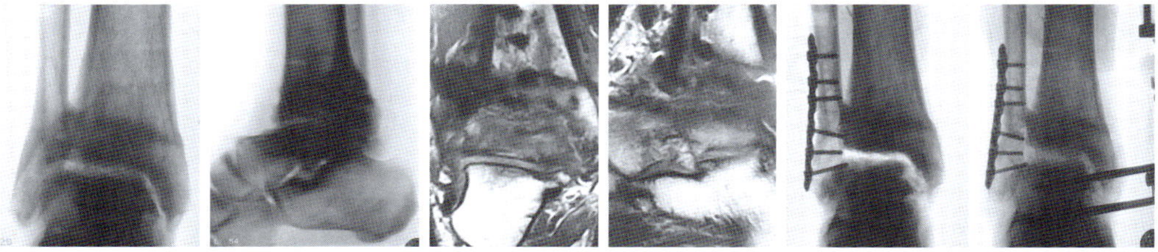

Figure 12 27-year-old male patient with early post-traumatic arosis at the tibio-tarsica, documented on X-rays and MRI. Cartilage repair is performed with bone marrow concentrate and scaffold, joint reconstruction with elongation of the fibula and subsequent arthrodiasis with external monoaxial fixator in distraction

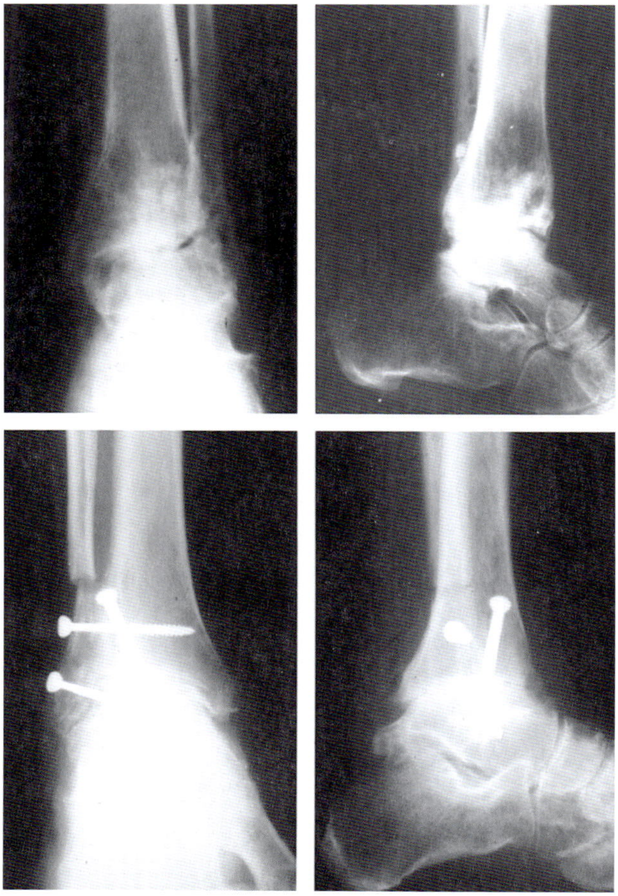

Figure 13 Top pre-operative X-rays in a 45-year-old patient with severe tibio-tarsal arthrosis. Below post-operative X-ray showing tibio-tarsal arthrodesis with screws

ve results even in the long term [24], arthrodesis is not a complication-free intervention; even in cases performed with correct indication and appropriate technique, pseudoarthrosis, consolidation defects, misalignments, and abnormalities of the march can occur [25,26]. A further complication is represented by the risk of developing arthrosis in the joints adjacent to the ankle [26] due to the important and increased stresses to which these are subjected, especially in young patients.

Starting from the 70s´, in an attempt to ensure greater functionality and thanks to the good results obtained in hip and knee prosthetics, the first models of tibio-tarsal prostheses were introduced. Thanks to the evolution of research, materials, and surgical techniques, the latest generation prostheses have shown encouraging results in the short and medium-term, associated with reduced complication rates and good recovery of joint function (fig. 14) [23].

However, to overcome some critical issues, especially in young and active patients, biological solutions have been developed that can reconstruct a native joint.

Transplantation of a bank joint to replace a damaged one is consolidated in orthopedic surgery. The use of frozen allografts has already known a wide diffusion in rescue surgery, both in the trauma and oncological fields. However, it is widely known that

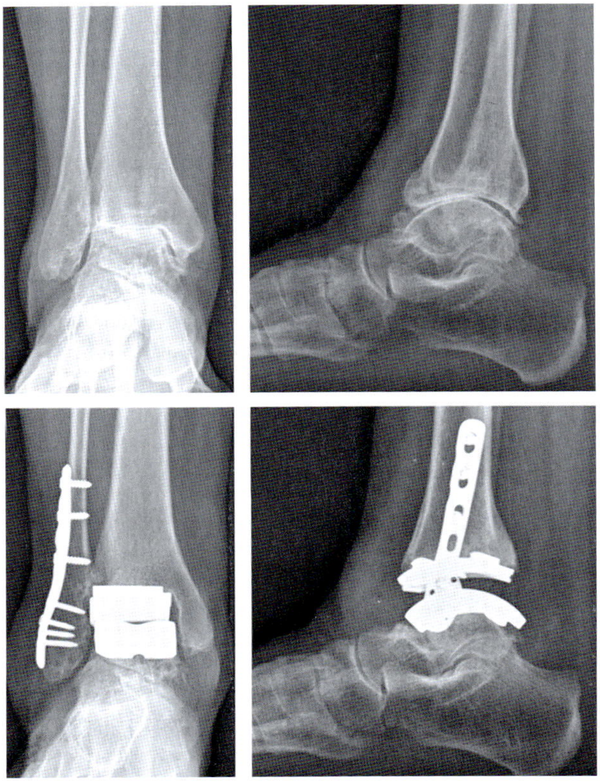

Figure 14 Top pre-operative X-rays in a 62-year-old female patient with severe tibio-tarsal arthrosis. Below post-operative X-ray showing ankle prostheses with lateral access (synthesized with peroneal plaque) 2 years after surgery

chondrocyte cells are not able to survive freezing, and the newly implanted joint is not equipped with viable cartilage and, given the large size of the transplant, is poorly reinhabited by the recipient [27].

The use of partial fresh transplants is also well documented. On the contrary total joint transplants are considerably less widespread and have shown valid and stable results over time, especially for small allografts [28].

New transplants have found wide application in knee surgery, partly at the ankle level (fig. 15) [28].

Fresh total osteochondral transplants are intended to be real biological prostheses, capable of offering vital cartilage capable of surviving transplantation and supported by a subchondral bone with a thin thickness (1cm) and therefore able to be progressively reinhabited by the recipient [29]. However, fresh transplantation is a technically complex procedure, and a large percentage of intraoperative and postoperative complications are reported [30-32].

Many factors contribute to determining the success in the use of biological prosthesis, including the surgical technique, the use of specific instru-

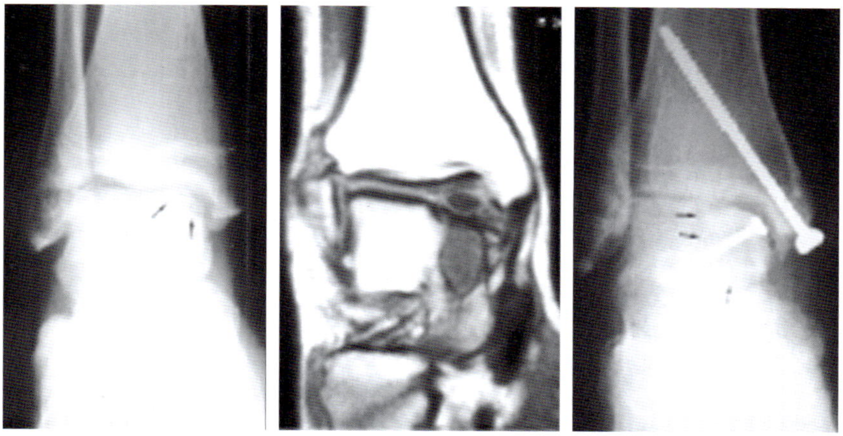

Figure 15 47-year-old male patient. On the left the X-ray shows severe medial astragal osteochondral lesion, confirmed by MRI in the center. The patient undergoes replacement with partial allograft, implanted by osteotomy of overturning the medial malleolus (then synthesized with screw)

ments, the postoperative protocol, and others still poorly known [33].

Patient candidates for total tibiotarsal allograft are ideally under 50 with post-traumatic bipolar osteoarthritis. Contraindications include osteoporosis, rheumatoid arthritis, infections, and malignant tumors. Malalignments of the lower limb, if any, must be corrected previously or in the same session of the allograft implant. In no case should the allograft be used to correct misalignment and shaped for this purpose.

Ankle transplants can be performed via double transperoneal lateral access (fig. 16) [33] or single anterior access (fig. 17) [34].

From the studies evaluated, ankle transplantation has proved to be an intervention capable of giving satisfactory results even at an extended follow-up. Although technically complex and not without complications, it is applicable

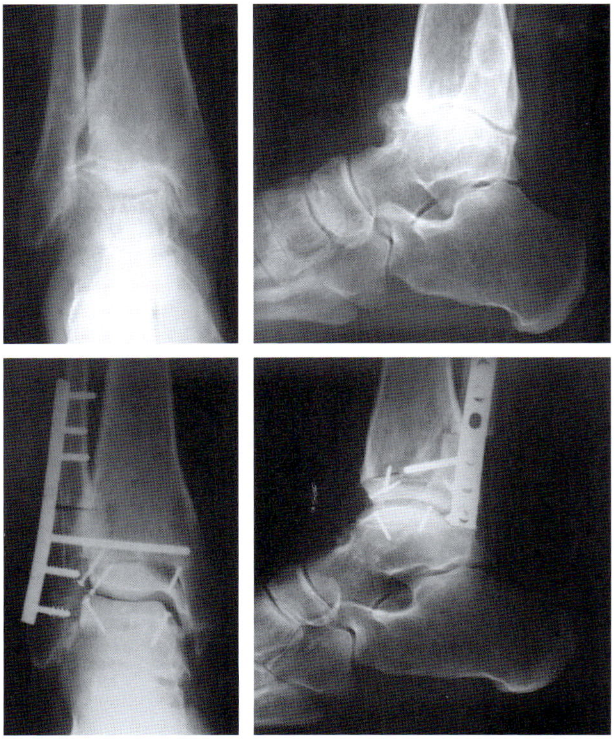

Figure 16 Top pre-operative X-rays in a 47-year-old male patient with severe tibio-tarsal arthrosis. Below post-operative X-rays showing fresh implanted bipolar total allograft with lateral access (synthesized with peroneal plaque)

with good results in selected indications. In the most recent published study [35], the survival of transplanted ankles exceeded 70% at 121 months. It was also noted that the improvement in the cases in general, including failures, was statistically significant ($p<0.0005$), but going to consider only the surviving cases, the final score was excellent or good in all cases, except two. This leads us to think that, despite the still significant percentage of failures, when the intervention is successful, it is perceived by the patient as a reasonable solution in most cases.

The main problems, excluding failures

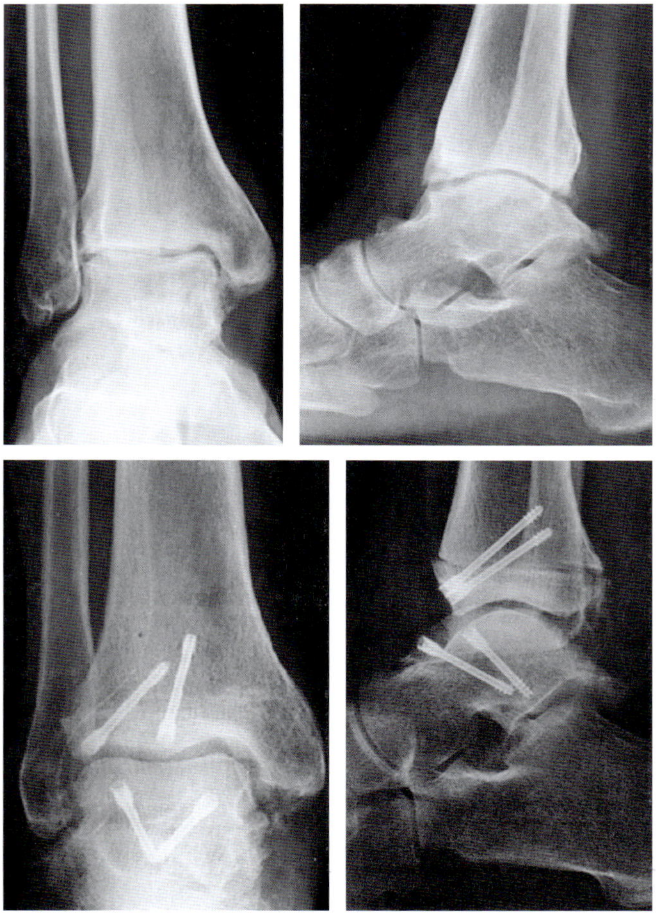

Figure 17 Top pre-operative X-rays in a 28-year-old male patient with severe tibio-tarsal arthrosis. Below post-operative X-rays showing fresh implanted bipolar total allograft with anterior access.

from malpositioning or fracture, seem to be related to progressive degeneration of the transplanted cartilage with consequent arthrosis and reduction of joint movement, although well-tolerated in most cases indolent.

Since the purpose of the intervention is not to obtain, even after some time, and expensive arthrodesis, it is evident, from the analysis of the literature, that some aspects deserve to be deepened.

In most organ transplants, a good match between donor and recipient of the blood type parameters AB0, Rh, and HLA is necessary. As for osteochondral transplants, this point has long been considered scarcely irrelevant, given the belief that joint tissue is immunoprivilegic. Underlying this belief is that the very dense matrix of articular cartilage is believed to prevent immune cells from recognizing antigens. However, allografts contain both a bone and a cartilage component, and although the cartilage was immunoprivilegiate, the bone is still immunogenic [36,37].

Regarding the correlations between the presence of antibodies to HLA and the clinical results of allograft at a follow-up of 10.6 years, the data were shown to be better in those patients who had a good HLA match [38].

Meehan et al. [39] described the follow-up of ankle transplants considering the HLA matching between donor and recipient. Six months after surgery, the presence of antibodies to HLA in the serum of all patients was detected. In a small series of failed cases, however, the analysis of the removed allografts showed the presence and colonization of CD4+, CD8+, and T cells [40].

The experience in using allograft as a biological alternative to the prosthesis in the forms of advanced arthrosis is worthy of being continued. However, it is necessary to focus on the critical issues and search for possible solutions to prevent the degeneration of the implanted cartilage.

Regenerative therapy in knee osteoarthritis

As with ankle osteoarthritis, one of the main problems in the treatment of arthritic injuries of the knee is the difficulty of reconstructing a native joint surface. This difficulty is all the greater, the more extensive the cartilage lesion.

The treatment algorithm is similar to what has already been described for the tibiotarsal joint.

In injuries arthrosis lesions up to grade 2 without misalignments, it is possible to perform regenerative treatments (fig. 18,19).

In grade 2/3 lesions, in the presence of misalignments, it is appropriate to resolve the defect on the frontal plane by osteotomies in relation to the pathological anatomy [41] (fig. 20).

In grade 3 lesions, as an alternative to traditional prosthetic replacement treatments, partial (fig. 21) or total (fig. 22,23) osteochondral transplants can be performed in relation to pathological anatomy. However, unlike partial allografts, the knee with total allografts did not achieve

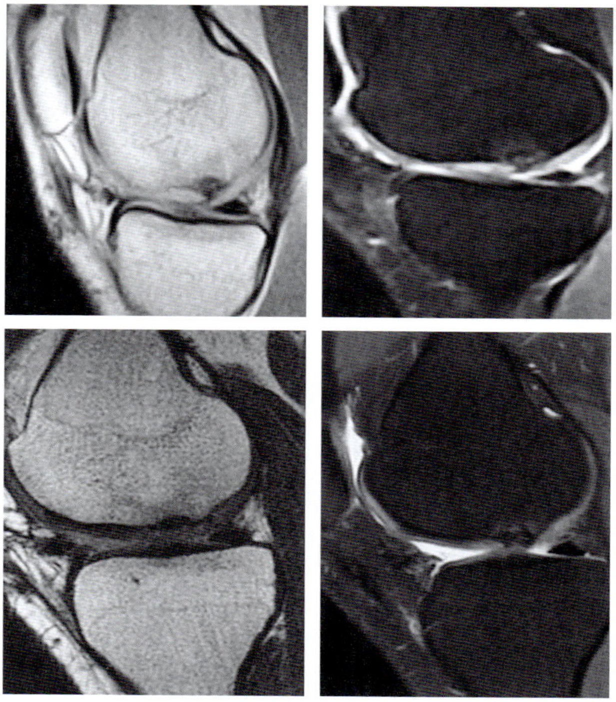

Figure 18 28-year-old female patient. At the top the MRI shows the osteochondral lesion of the femoral condyle. Below the MRI after 12 months shows the almost total filling of the defect after arthroscopic chondral repair by reclamation and implantation of scaffolds with concentrate of concentrated autologous bone marrow mononuclear cells

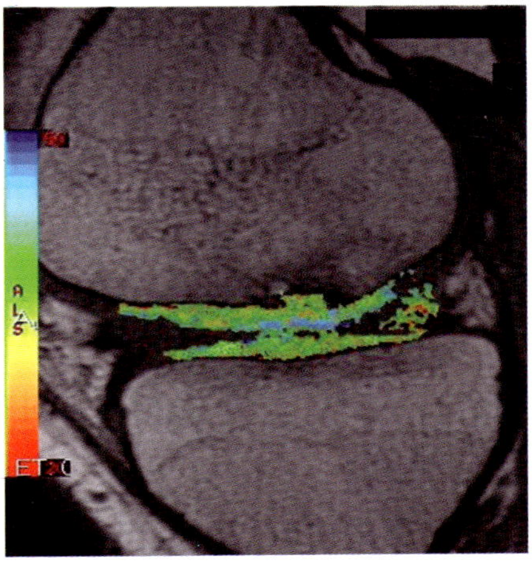

Figure 19 Female patient aged 28 years (same as figure 18). MRI T2 mapping 2 years after arthroscopic chondral repair by reclamation and implantation of scaffolds with concentrate of concentrated autologous bone marrow mononuclear cells. The examination shows a good regenerated with characteristics like hyaline cartilage in terms of hydration

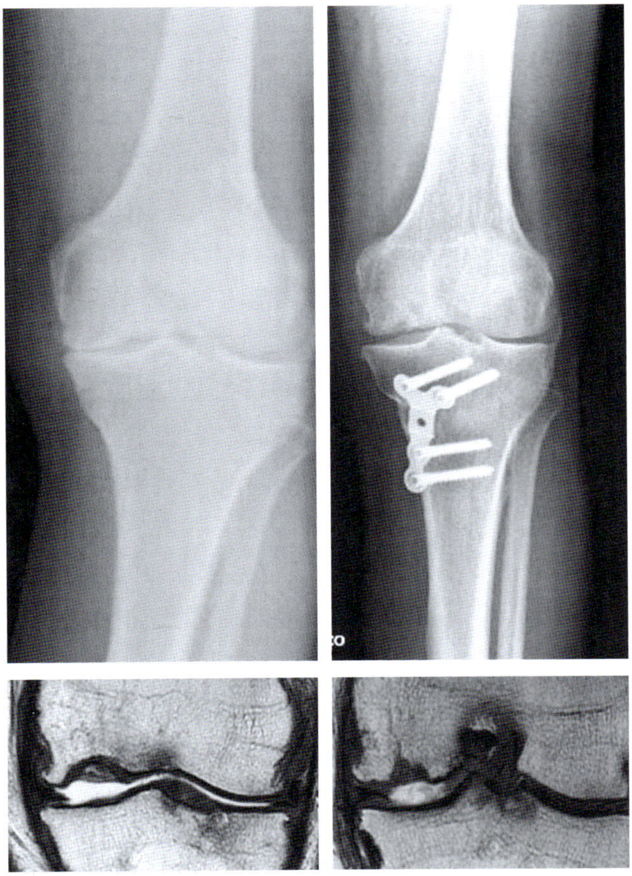

Figure 20 46-year-old male patient with varus knee. At the top left the pre-operative x-rays under load. The patient undergoes osteotomy in plus with bank bone wedge grafting, synthesized with plaque and screws (RX at the top right) and chondral repair of the medial femoral condyle by reclamation and implantation of scaffolds with concentrate of bone marrow mononuclear cells. Lower left MRI in the pre-operative showing extensive chondral lesion. Bottom right MRI 12 months after surgery

the same good results as the ankle, probably due to the high amount of soft parts [42].

Conclusions

The evolution of surgical techniques in treating arthritic lesions, together

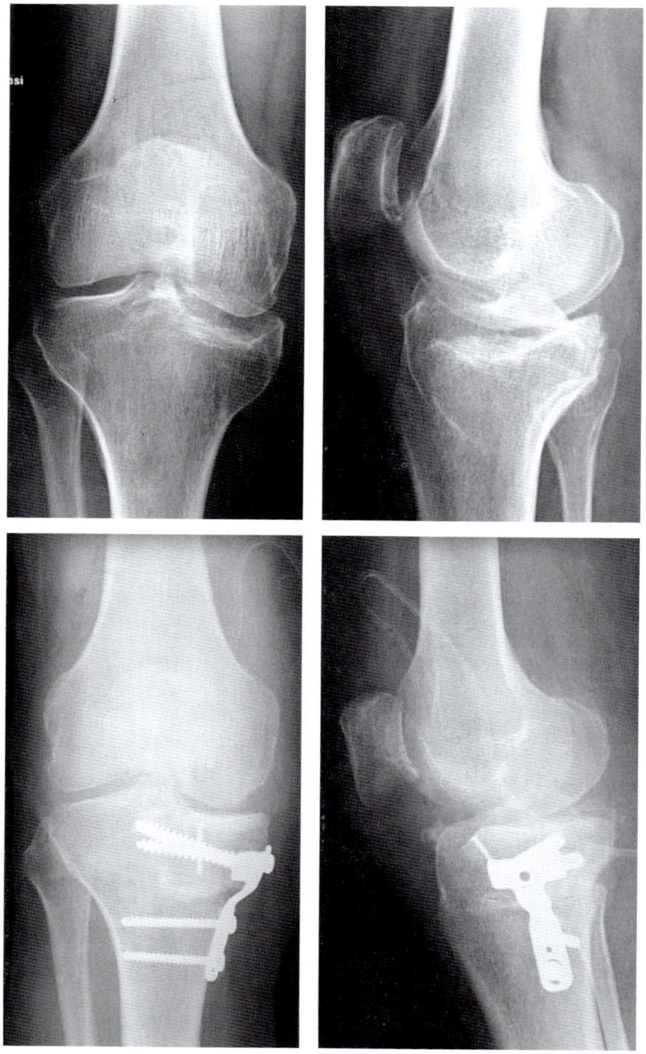

Figura 21 Top RX in 2 projections of the right knee under load in male 50 years, with severe defect of the medial tibial plate in septic arthritis outcomes. The patient undergoes replacement of the medial tibial plate with partial allograft, synthesized with plaque and screws (RX below)

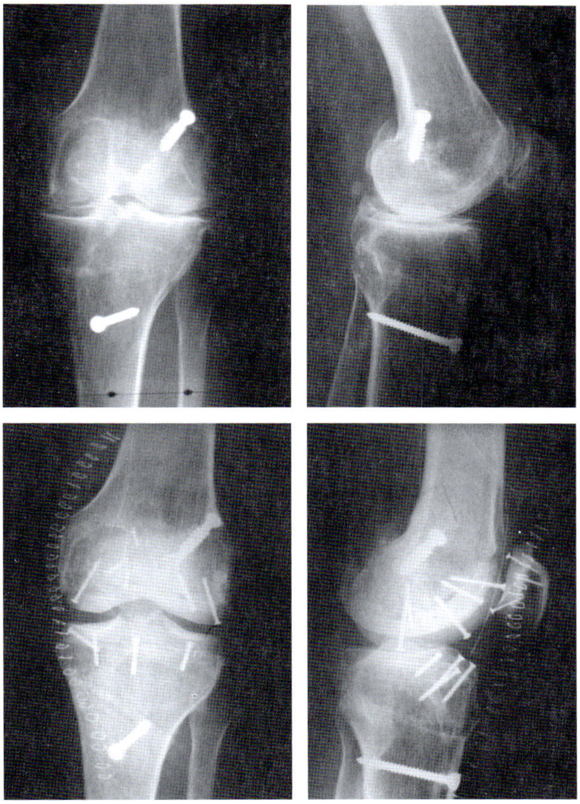

Figura 22 Top RX in 2 projections of the right knee under load in 34-year-old male, with severe post-traumatic osteoarthritis of the knee. The patient undergoes total joint replacement with fresh bipolar allograft, synthesized with screws (RX below)

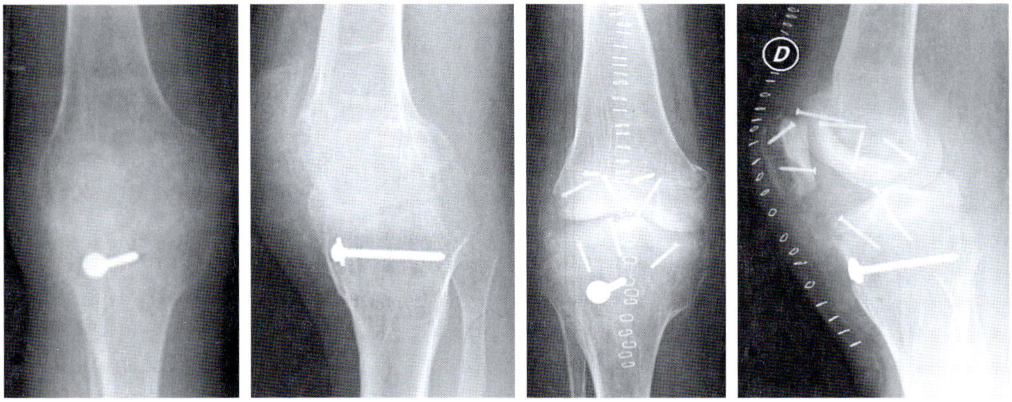

Figura 23 Left RX in anteroposterior and lateral projection in 27-year-old male patient with arthrodesis of the left knee. The patient undergoes dysarthrodesis and implantation of fresh bipolar allograft, synthesized with screws (RX below) (43)

with the most recent research achievements, has led to the development of methods increasingly attentive to biology and based on tissue regeneration, especially in young and active patients. The "One-Step" technique by implanting scaffolds with autologous bone marrow mononuclear cell concentrate has shown encouraging results in young and selected patients. It represents an emerging option in treating early osteoarthritis lesions of both the ankle and knee to delay or avoid prosthetic interventions to the joint involved.

Biological joint reconstructions have already offered a good percentage of satisfactory results, both in the ankle and knee.

Fresh total allograft from a donor represents a biological alternative to ankle prosthesis or arthrodesis in young and selected patients.

Unlike partial allografts, the same results were not obtained in the knee with the total allograft due to the high amount of soft parts.

Therefore further immunological research is therefore needed to understand the reasons for the failures.

References

1. Hangody L, Vasarhelyi G, Hangody LR, et al. Autologous osteochondral grafting - technique and long-termresults. Injury 2008;39(Suppl 1):S32-9.
2. Ferruzzi A, Buda R, Faldini C, et al. Autologous chondrocyte implantation in the knee joint: open compared with arthroscopic technique. Comparison at a minimum follow-up of five years. J Bone Joint Surg Am 2008;90(Suppl 4):90-101.
3. Marcacci M, Kon E, Delcogliano M, et al. Arthroscopic autologous osteochondral grafting for cartilage defects of the knee: prospective study results at a minimum 7-year followup. Am J Sports Med 2007;35:2014-21.
4. Gobbi A, Bathan L. Biological approaches for cartilage repair. J Knee Surg 2009;22:36-44.
5. Peterson L, Brittberg M, Kiviranta I, et al. Autologous chondrocyte transplantation. Biomechanics and long-term durability. Am J Sports Med 2002;30:2-12.
6. Magnussen RA, Dunn WR, Carey JL, et al. Treatment of focal articular cartilage defects in the knee: a systematic review. Clin Orthop Relat Res 2008;466:952-62.
7. Oreffo ROC, Cooper C, Mason C, et al. Mesenchymal stem cells: lineage, plasticity, and skeletal therapeutic potential. Stem Cell Reviews 2005;1:169-78.
8. Buda R, Vannini F, Cavallo M, et al. One-step bone marrowderived cell transplantation in talarosteochondral lesions: mid-term results. Joints 2014;1:102-7.

9. Buda R, Vannini F, Castagnini F, Cavallo M, Ruffilli A, Ramponi L, Pagliazzi G, Giannini S. Regenerative treatment in osteochondral lesions of the talus: autologous chondrocyte implantation versus one-step bone marrow derived cells transplantation. Int Orthop. 2015 May;39(5):893-900.
10. Giannini S, Buda R, Battaglia M, et al. One-step repair in talar osteochondral lesions: 4-year clinical results and t2-mapping capability in outcome prediction. Am J Sports Med 2013;41:511-8.
11. Cavallo M, Sayyed-Hosseinian SH, Parma A, Buda R, Mosca M, Giannini S. Combination of High Tibial Osteotomy and Autologous Bone Marrow Derived Cell Implantation in Early Osteoarthritis of Knee: A Preliminary Study. Arch Bone Jt Surg. 2018 Mar;6(2):112-118.
12. Buda R, Castagnini F, Cavallo M, Ramponi L, Vannini F, Giannini S. "One-step" bone marrow-derived cells transplantation and joint debridement for osteochondral lesions of the talus in ankle osteoarthritis: clinical and radiological outcomes at 36 months. Arch Orthop Trauma Surg. 2016 Jan;136(1):107-16.
13. Van Dijk, CN; Verhagen RA; Tol, JL: Arthroscopy for problems after ankle fracture. J. Bone Joint Surg. 79.B:280-284, 19970.
14. Galois L, Freyria AM, Herbage D, Mainard D. Cartilage tissue engineering: state-of-the-art and future approaches. Pathol Biol Paris 2005; 53(10): 590-598.
15. Oreffo RO, Cooper C, Mason C, Clements M. Mesenchymal stem cells: lineage, plasticity, and skeletal therapeutic potential. Stem Cell Rev 2005; 1(2): 169-178.
16. Giannini S., Buda R. Ankle arthroscopy. Technique and therapeutic addresses. Timaeus 2011.
17. Pardue EL, Ibrahim S, Ramamurthi A. Role of hyaluronan in angiogenesis and its utility to angiogenic tissue engineering. Organogenesis 2008; 4: 203-214.
18. Giannini S, Buda R, Vannini F, Cavallo M, Grigolo B. One-step bone marrow-derived cell transplantation in talar osteochondral lesions. Clin Orthop Relat Res. 2009 Dec;467(12):3307-20.
19. Giannini S, Buda R, Cavallo M, et al. Cartilage repair evolution in post-traumatic osteochondral lesions of the talus: from open field autologous chondrocyte to bone-marrow-derived cells transplantation. Injury 2010;41:1196-1203.
20. Baldassarri M, Perazzo L, Ricciarelli M, et al. Regenerative treatment of osteochondral lesions of distal tibial plafond. Eur J Orthop Surg Traumatol 2018;28:1199-1207. doi: 10.1007/ s00590-018-2161-7. Epub 2018 Feb 23.
21. Zgonis T, Stapleton J, Roukis T. Use of the Taylor spatial frame for arthrodiastasis of the ankle joint. Techniques in foot and ankle surgery 2007. 6:201-207.
22. Magnan, B., et al. "Arthrodiatasis in degenerative ankle disease. Valid solution?." Archive of Orthopedics and Rheumatology 121.4 (2010): 25-27.

23. Giannini S, Buda R, Faldini C, Vannini F, Romagnoli M, Grandi G, Bevoni R The treatment of severe posttraumatic arthritis of the ankle joint. The Journal of Bone and Joint Surgery American. 2007 Oct;89 Suppl 3:15-28.
24. R. H. Thomas and T. R. Daniels. Ankle arthritis. Journal of Bone and Joint Surgery A, vol. 85, no. 5, pp. 923–936, 2003.
25. Takakura Y, Tanaka Y, Sugimoto K, Akiyama K, Tamai S. Long-term results of arthrodesis for osteoarthritis of the ankle. Clin Orthop Relat Res. 1999 Apr;(361):178-85.
26. Coester LM, Saltzman CL, Leupold J, Pontarelli W. Long-term results following ankle ar-throdesis for post-traumatic arthritis. J Bone Joint Surg Am. 2001 Feb;83-A(2):219-28.
27. Czitrom AA, Keating S, Gross AE. The viability of articular cartilage in fresh osteochondral allografts after clinical transplantation. The Journal of Bone and Joint Surgery American. 1990;72(4):574-581.
28. Gross AE, McKee NH, Pritzker KP, Langer F. Reconstruction of skeletal deficits at the knee. A comprehensive osteochondral transplant program. Clinical Orthopaedics and Related Research. 1983;(174):96-106.
29. Tontz WL Jr, Bugbee WD, Brage ME. Use of allografts in the management of ankle arthritis. Foot And Ankle Clinics. 2003;8(2):361-373.
30. Kim CW, Jamali A, Tontz W Jr, Convery FR, Brage ME, Bugbee W. Treatment of post-traumatic ankle arthrosis with bipolar tibiotalar osteochondral shell allografts. Foot & Ankle International. 2002;23(12):1091-102.
31. Meehan R, McFarlin S, Bugbee W, Brage M. Fresh ankle osteochondral allograft transplantation for tibiotalar joint arthritis. Foot & Ankle International. 2005 Oct;26(10):793-802.
32. Jeng CL, Kadakia A, White KL, Myerson MS. Fresh osteochondral total ankle allograft transplantation for the treatment of ankle arthritis. Foot & Ankle International. 2008 Jun;29(6):554-60.
33. Giannini S, Buda R, Grigolo B, Bevoni R, Di Caprio F, Ruffilli A, Cavallo M, Desando G, Vannini F. Bipolar fresh osteochondral allograft of the ankle. Foot & Ankle International 2010 Jan;31(1):38-46.
34. Giannini S, Buda R, Pagliazzi G, Ruffilli A, Cavallo M, Baldassarri M, Vannini F. Survivorship of bipolar fresh total osteochondral ankle allograft. Foot & Ankle International 2014 Mar;35(3):243-51. Epub 2014 Jan 8.
35. Giannini S, Mazzotti A, Vannini F. Bipolar fresh total osteochondral allograft in the ankle: Is it a successful long-term solution? Injury. 2017. Jul;48(7):1319-1324.
36. Bonfiglio M, Jeter WS and Smith C: The immune concept: its relation to bone transplantation. Annals of the New York Academy of Sciences. 1955; 59: 417.
37. Chalmers J: Transplantation immunity in bone homografting. The Journal of Bone and Joint Surgery British. 1959; 41B: 160.

38. Friedlaender GE, Strong DM, Tomford WW, Mankin HJ. Long-term follow-up of patients with osteochondral allografts: a correlation between immunologic responses and clinical outcome. Orthopedic Clinics of North America. 1999;30(4):583-588.
39. Meehan R, McFarlin S, Bugbee W, Brage M. Fresh ankle osteochondral allograft transplantation for tibiotalar joint arthritis. Foot & Ankle International. 2005 Oct;26(10):793-802.
40. Pomajzl RJ, Baker EA, Baker KC, et al. Case series with histopathologic and radiographic analyses following failure of fresh osteochondral allografts of the talus. Foot & Ankle International. 2016;37(9):958-967.
41. Cavallo M, Sayyed-Hosseinian SH, Parma A, Buda R, Mosca M, Giannini S. Combination of High Tibial Osteotomy and Autologous Bone Marrow Derived Cell Implantation in Early Osteoarthritis of Knee: A Preliminary Study. Arch Bone Jt Surg. 2018 Mar;6(2):112-118.
42. Giannini S, Buda R, Ruffilli A, Pagliazzi G, Ensini A, Grigolo B, Desando G, Vannini F. Failures in bipolar fresh osteochondral allograft for the treatment of end-stage knee osteoarthritis. Knee Surg Sports Traumatol Arthrosc. 2015 Jul;23(7):2081-9.
43. Giannini S, Buda R, Ruffilli A, Pagliazzi G, Vannini F. Total femoral and tibial osteochondral allograft for remobilizing a knee after arthrodesis. Knee Surg Sports Traumatol Arthrosc. 2013 Dec;21(12):2784-9.

CHAPTER 8

GROWTH DRIVERS IN REGENERATIVE APPLICATIONS

Brunella Grigolo
Head of SSD Laboratory RAMSES, IRCCS Rizzoli Orthopaedic Institute, Bologna

Introduction

Regenerative medicine represents "an interdisciplinary field that applies the principles of engineering and life sciences towards developing biological substitutes that restore, maintain or improve tissue function" [1]. The protagonists of this therapeutic strategy are cells (e.g., adult, mesenchymal), natural and/or synthetic biomaterials, and growth factors (fig. 1). In the orthopedic field, the study of this innovative technology has long involved surgeons and researchers in realizing its use to repair and/or replace damaged tissues of the musculoskeletal system.

Injuries due to trauma are very frequent and represent a significant economic impact on the national health service. The multiple surgical proce-

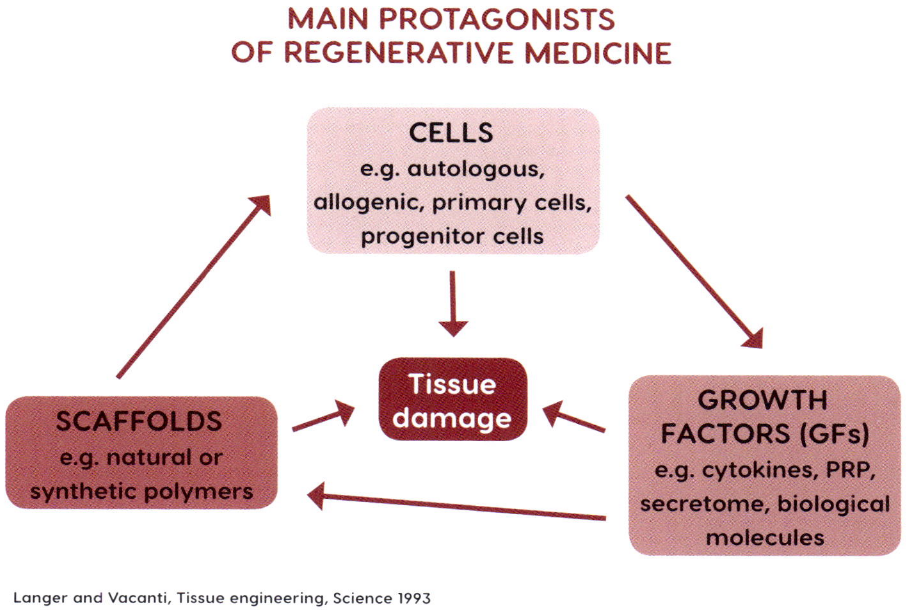

Figure 1 In the image, the main protagonists of regenerative medicine. Cells (adult, mesenchymal), biomaterials (natural or synthetic) growth factors (cytokines, platelet-rich plasma, secretome, other biological molecules).

dures often required are associated with patient morbidity and reduced quality of life. Tissue engineering is an interdisciplinary field that applies the principles of engineering and life sciences to the development of biological substitutes to restore, maintain or improve the function of damaged tissues and organs. In this field of research, knowledge of cell biology, engineering, materials science, and surgery is therefore merged to build new functional tissues through the combination of cells, biomaterials, and growth factors. The application of this therapeutic strategy for the regeneration of tissues of the musculoskeletal system has represented an important turning point in the clinical approach of the treatment of numerous diseases of the musculoskeletal system.

Growth factors (GFs)

Biological agents represent an emerging treatment modality for a variety of musculoskeletal pathologies. These agents include natural growth factors and anti-inflammatory mediators that can accelerate tissue healing and recovery. They can act through various mechanisms, including increased angiogenesis, matrix synthesis and remodeling, cell recruitment, and modulation of inflammatory markers and metalloproteinases.

The possible role played by GFs in pain reduction and tissue regeneration has generated a growing interest in their possible therapeutic use in patients with musculoskeletal injuries. However, significant clinical data on the actual potential to support their regular use are still lacking. In recent years, discoveries, combined with knowledge of the importance and role of growth factors for tissue engineering, have been further developed and deepened [2]. The term "growth factor" (often used in the English form "growth factor" – GF – or with the generic term of "growth factor") refers to proteins naturally secreted by cells and essential for regenerative processes. Growth factors facilitate and promote the regeneration of new tissues by interacting with specific transmembrane receptors and regulating protein synthesis within cells. Binding to the specific growth factor receptor specifically stimulates cell signal transduction pathways that trigger cell migration, survival, adhesion, proliferation, growth, and differentiation. Their ability to influence protein synthesis and cellular interactions make them a key tool in controlling stem cell differentiation; for example, Bone Morphogenic Protein -2 (BMP-2) for the regulation of osteogenesis, Vascular Endothelial Growth Factor (VEGF) for angiogenesis, and Transforming Growth Factor-beta (TGF-beta) for chondrogenesis and many others. GFs have been classified into several major families, mainly TGF-β, Fibroblast Growth Factors (FGFs), Platelet-Derived Growth Factors (PDGFs), and Nuclear Factor-KappaB (NF-kappa β). The superfamily of TGF-β is the largest one, comprising the main groups of polypeptide morphogens.

This family is divided into two subgroups. The first of these subgroups, which includes GFs such as TGF-β, exhibits functions in cell adhesion, growth, cytoskeletal organization, survival, migration, proliferation, differentiation, chemotaxis, and activation of many cells of the immune system during the development of multicellular organisms.

The other group of the TGF-β superfamily is BMPs. However, only a part of these (BMP-2, BMP-4, BMP-6, BMP-7, and BMP-9) significantly affects bone formation. BMP-1 is not part of the TGF-β family but belongs to the metalloproteinase family.

Although growth factors have great potential to stimulate cartilage or bone repair, only a limited number of treatments have been approved by government regulatory agencies for clinical use. The bone morphogenetic activity was first described in 1965, but only in 2001 and 2002 two protein biotherapies, using morphogenetic proteins, such as BMP-2 and BMP-7 were approved by the US Food and Drug Administration (FDA) for use in the treatment of pseudoarthrosis of long bones, exposed fractures of the tibia and spinal fusion.

Current off-label use includes foot and ankle arthrodesis procedures, treatment of high-risk fractures, and pseudoarthrosis. Among the commercially available recombinant factors we have human BMPs (rhBMP) and, approved for clinical use, there are Infuse (Medtronic Sofamor Danek, Memphis, TN, USA), rhBMP-2 and OP-1 Putty (Stryker Biotech, Hopkinton, MA, USA), and rhBMP-7.

However, despite the literature supports the potential of BMPs, their use in fracture healing has significantly decreased compared with other orthobiological ones. This is because they are expensive molecules. Some morbidities are associated with their use, including excessive heterotopic bone formation (given in particular the tendency of BMP to penetrate the surrounding soft tissues), the hidden potential for carcinogenesis, renal and hepatic insufficiency, and compartment syndrome. At this time, the indications for BMP use in sports medicine outside the treatment of atrophic non-unions are unclear and require further investigation [3,4].

Platelet-Rich Plasma (PRP)

Platelet-rich plasma represents an inexpensive source for obtaining many GFs in physiological proportion and has already been widely applied as a carrier of GFs in different fields of medicine (sports medicine, orthopedics, dermatology, ophthalmology, plastic and maxillofacial surgery, neurosurgery, urology, and cardiothoracic surgery) for its property of promoting regeneration of tissues even in those with low healing potential [5]. PRP can be defined as a blood derivative in which platelets have a very high concentration (fig. 2).

Platelets have demonstrated osteoinductive properties precisely because they are rich in important growth factors. In particular, alpha platelet granules contain and release numerous growth factors, including PDGF, TGF-β 1, VEGF, Epidermal Growth Factor (EGF), Fibroblast Growth Factor (FGF), and Insulin-like Growth Factors (IGF). The widespread use of PRP in orthopedics applies to bone regeneration, where PRP has shown positive results. An example, PRP in-

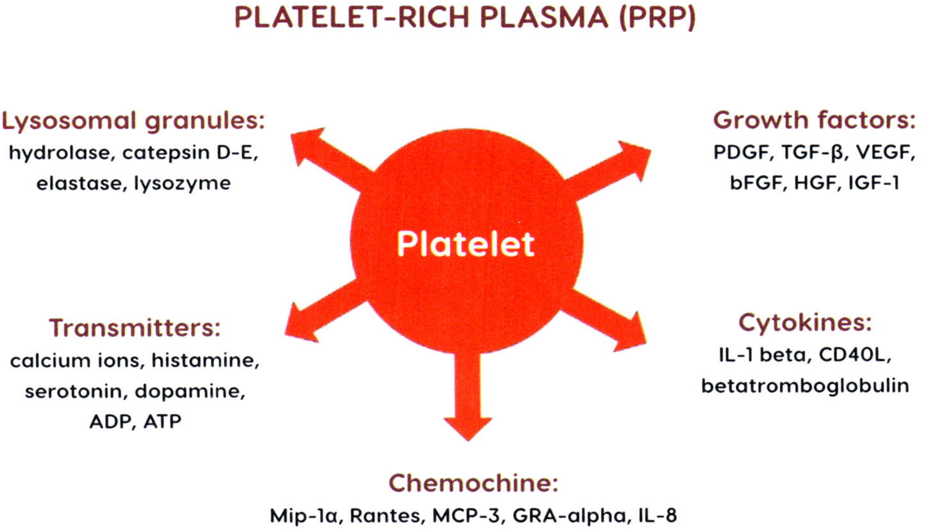

Figure 2 Platelet-Rich Plasma (PRP) has high concentration of molecules that have proven to be active against bone and cartilage

jected at the fracture site of a lack of atrophic consolidation of long bone led to 87% union 4 months after treatment. A comparison between the use of PRP and an intramedullary nail in the non-union repair of long bones showed in the first case a healing rate of about 93% compared to 80% of the other group. However, despite the widespread use of PRP for the treatment of various tissues of the musculoskeletal system, the exact biological composition and its effects on healing remain to be clarified. One of the main problems with PRP is that there are numerous preparation protocols, which result in different preparations that are injected into the patient [6,7].

The secretome of Mesenchymal Stem Cells

Over the years, mesenchymal stem cells (MSCs) in regenerative medicine have replaced differentiated adult cells due to their many advantages. MSCs are multipotent cells present in adult bone marrow and, as such, have the ability to differentiate into mesenchymal tissue lines, including cartilage, bone, fat. MSCs represent a promising cellular source for the regeneration of tissues of the musculoskeletal system as they are easily obtainable in large numbers and expandable in vitro. Some limitations to their application are related to the potential malignant transformation due to their multipotency, the possible transmission of pathogens, and their survival and home at the site of injury once implanted. Although it was initially believed that the potential of MSCs to differentiate into various cell types played their main therapeutic effect, it later emerged that their major role in this regard is represented by their trophic, paracrine, and immunomodulatory functions [8] (fig. 3).

MSCs secrete bioactive molecules that

- inhibit apoptosis by limiting the area of injury;
- inhibit the formation of fibrosis or scarring at the sites of injury;
- stimulate angiogenesis and a new blood supply;
- stimulate mitosis of tissue-specific progenitors.

MSCs also secrete immunomodulatory agents that deactivate T cell surveillance and chronic inflammatory processes. By this observation, the use of secretome for tissue regeneration has therefore been increasingly hypothesized [9]. The use of this compound is based on its composition rich in trophic factors (chemokines, cytokines, hormones, and lipid mediators) with paracrine effects on the cells of the local microenvironment. Among GFs, IGF, VEGF, TGF β 1, and Hepatocyte Growth Factor (HGF) can affect angiogenesis and resident cell migration.

The soluble factors contained in the secretome could then initiate regenerative signaling events without cells. The therapeutic effect of this biological product in musculoskeletal diseases is an important frontier novelty of regenerative medicine and is still little

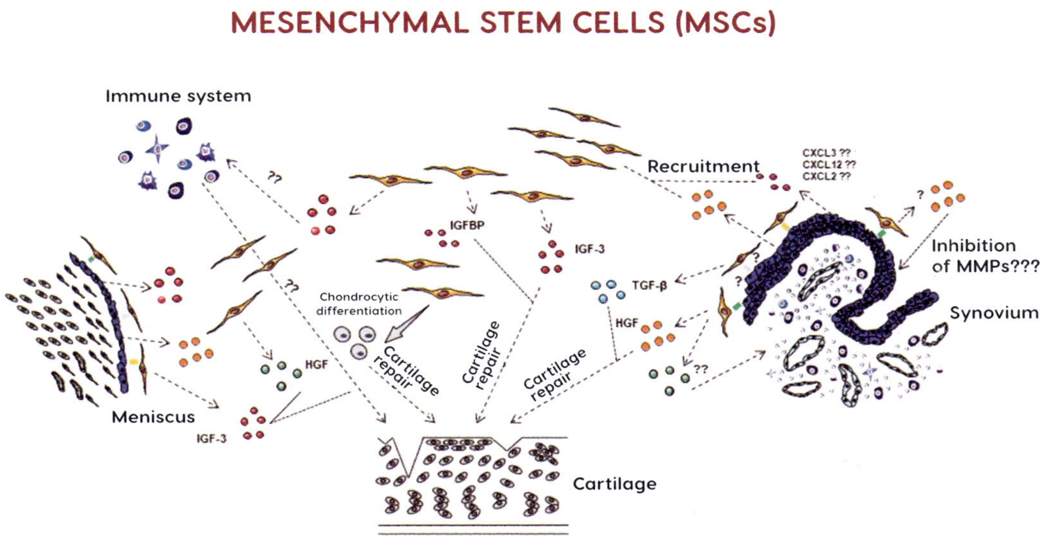

Figure 3 Mesenchymal stem cells (MSCs) and their secretome. In the image, the possible targets of therapy with mesenchymal cells and actions of the molecules present in the secretome on the various components of the joint

studied and used. Its use could eliminate the negative aspects of the use of cells and, at the same time, could help concentrate paracrine factors at physiological levels at the site of the injury. However, many studies provide clear evidence for the power of the factors secreted by MSC in the mediation of tissue repair and regeneration, the precise mechanisms by which MSCs act paracrine are not yet fully understood.

Extracellular vesicles (ECVs)

It has been recognized that the paracrine action of MSCs is not limited to the production of soluble factors but that these cells, like many others, are able to produce a large number of extracellular vesicles (EVs) [10]. The latter are involved in intercellular communication by releasing mRNAs and proteins; they also have anti-apoptotic, antifibrotic, pro-angiogenic, and anti-inflammatory effects. EVs released by tissue-damaged cells can reprogram the stem cell phenotype by making them acquire tissue-specific characteristics by releasing specific mRNAs and/or microRNAs. EVs produced by MSCs recruited from circulation or resident can reprogram tissue-damaged cells by providing mRNAs and/or miRNAs that induce de-differentiation, production of soluble paracrine mediators, and initiation of the cell cycle of these cells by promoting tissue regeneration [11] (fig. 4).

New biological molecules for bone regeneration: hydrogen sulfide

Recently, numerous biological molecules have been shown to stimulate

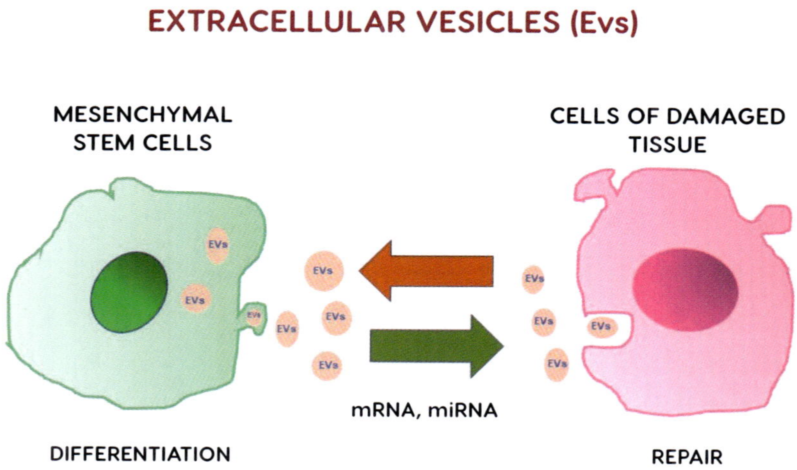

Figure 4 Extracellular Vesicles (EVs). Schematic representation of EVs-mediated mechanisms through which bidirectional exchanges occur between mesenchymal stem cells and damaged cells. The transfer of genetic information from the latter induces the differentiation of resident stem cells with tissue-specific phenotypes. RNAs derived from stem cells can, in turn, induce de-differentiation and resumption of the cell cycle and activate the regenerative process in damaged cells.
miRNA= microRNA

the regeneration of tissues of the musculoskeletal system, and their use in regenerative medicine could pave the way for new therapeutic uses [12]. Among these, it has been seen how hydrogen sulfide (H_2S), a gas present both in the environment and in living organisms and known to occupational medicine mainly for its toxicity, typical of the petrochemical environment, actually possesses the ability to modulate important biological functions. In fact, in the skeleton, the role of H_2S has been studied only in very recent times, revealing regulatory effects of great interest. For example, H_2S exerts a protective effect against oxidative damage in osteoblasts in bone cells. A study carried out on animal models showed that H_2S plays a fundamental role in the differentiation of stem cells in the osteogenic sense through the modulation of calcium channels. In our laboratory, we have demonstrated how the anti-oxidant effect of H_2S on osteoclasts (cells responsible for bone loss) determines a marked inhibition of the differentiation and function of these cells, suggesting a possible therapeutic use of H_2S in pathologies such as osteoporosis (fig. 5). Using mouse models of postmenopausal osteoporosis, it has been observed that an administration of H_2S by pharmacological route (using drugs capable of releasing H_2S in biological fluids) is able to completely prevent the loss of bone mass typical of osteoporosis through a mechanism that determines a stimulation of osteoblasts to form new bone tissue [13]. In the same study, it was shown that osteoporosis is associated with a marked decrease in plasma levels of H_2S, suggesting for the first time that a deficiency of the latter could play a facilitating role in the onset phase of the disease. Therefore, "exogenous" administration of H_2S would help restore H_2S levels in patients who would otherwise be deficient due to the pathological condition in which they are located.

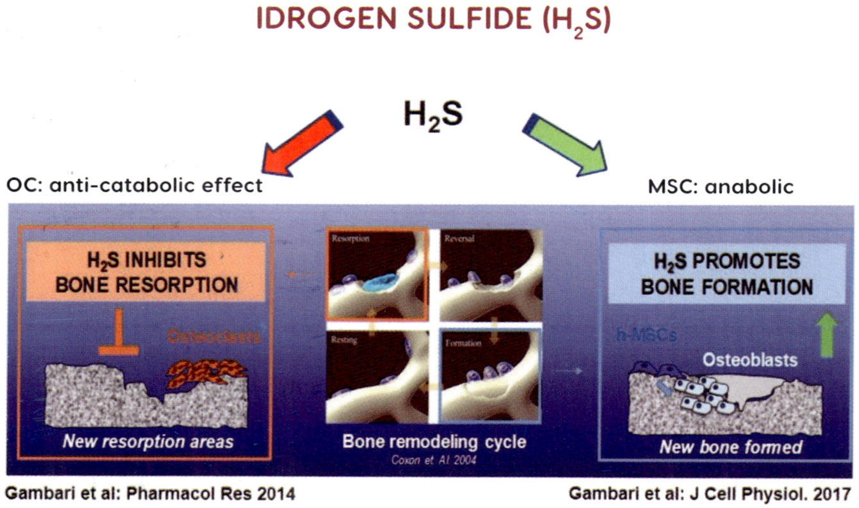

Figure 5 Hydrogen sulfide (H_2S). The anti-oxidant effect of H_2S on osteoclasts (cells responsible for bone loss) determines a marked inhibition of the differentiation and function of these cells and stimulation of anabolism by MSCs, suggesting a possible therapeutic use of H_2S in diseases such as osteoporosis

Conclusions

The use of bioactive factors in the clinical management of damage to the musculoskeletal system has progressed considerably in recent years. Innovative biological and engineering technologies have significantly improved the effectiveness and efficiency of these factors. Recent advances in the understanding of the mechanism of action of GFs and the results of studies carried out so far point to a fundamental role in the future of regenerative medicine.

References

1. Langer R, JP Vacanti. Tissue engineering. Science 1993 May 14;260(5110):920-6.
2. Subbiah R, Guldberg RE. Materials Science and Design Principles of Growth Factor Delivery Systems in Tissue Engineering and Regenerative Medicine. Adv Health Mater. 2019 Jan;8(1): e 1801000.
3. Atienza-Roca P, Cui X, Hooper GJ, Woodfield TBF, Lim KS. Growth Factor Delivery Systems for Tissue Engineering and

Regenerative Medicine. Adv Exp Med Biol. 2018;1078:245-269.

4. Sinclair KL, Mafi P, Mafi R, Khan WS. The Use of Growth Factors and Mesenchymal Stem Cells in Orthopaedics: In particular, their use in Fractures and Non-Unions: A Systematic Review. Curr Stem Cell Res Ther. 2017;12(4):312-325.
5. Anitua E, Sánchez M, Nurden AT, et al. New insights into and novel applications for platelet-rich fibrin therapies. Trends Biotechnol. 24:227–34, 2006.
6. Sampson S, Gerhardt M, Mandelbaum B. Platelet rich plasma injection grafts for musculoskeletal injuries: a review. Curr Rev Musculoskelet Med. 1:165–74, 2008.
7. Gentile P, Garcovich S. Systematic Review-The Potential Implications of Different Platelet-Rich Plasma (PRP) Concentrations in Regenerative Medicine for Tissue Repair. Int J Mol Sci. 2020 Aug 9;21(16):5702.
8. Murphy MB, Moncivais K, Caplan AI. Mesenchymal stem cells: environmentally responsive therapeutics for regenerative medicine. Exp Mol Med. 2013, 15;45(11) :e54.
9. Veronesi F, Borsari V, Sartori M, Orciani M, Mattioli-Belmonte M, Fini M. The use of cell conditioned medium for musculoskeletal tissue regeneration. J Cell Physiol. 2018 Jun;233(6):4423-4442
10. D'Arrigo D, Roffi A, Cucchiarini M, Moretti M, Candrian C, Filardo G. Secretome and Extracellular Vesicles as New Biological Therapies for Knee Osteoarthritis: A Systematic Review.J Clin Med. 2019 Nov 4;8(11):1867.
11. Rani S, Ryan AE, Griffin MD, Ritter T. Mesenchymal Stem Cell-derived Extracellular Vesicles: Toward Cell-free Therapeutic Applications Mol Ther. 2015 May;23(5):812-823.
12. Gambari L, Grigolo B, Grassi F. Hydrogen Sulfide in Bone Tissue Regeneration and Repair: State of the Art and New Perspectives. Int J Mol Sci. 2019 Oct 22;20(20):5231.
13. Grassi F, Tyagi AM, Calvert JW, Gambari L, Walker LD, Yu M, Robinson J, Li JY, Lisignoli G, Vaccaro C, Adams J, Pacifici R. Hydrogen Sulfide Is a Novel Regulator of Bone Formation Implicated in the Bone Loss Induced by Estrogen Deficiency. J Bone Miner Res. 2016 May;31(5):949-63.

CHAPTER 9

MESENCHYMAL STEM CELLS, TISSUE OF ORIGIN AND PECULIARITIES

Enrico Lucarelli, Barbara Dozza

Biologist, Laboratory of Orthopedic Pathology and Osteoarticular Tissue Regeneration, IRCCS Rizzoli Orthopaedic Institute, Bologna

Introduction

Stem cells remain immature until a stimulus intervenes that causes them to differentiate into specialized cells to fulfill a specific function in organs or tissues. They are cells that have the potential to develop into many of the body's cell types both during the first months of the individual's life and during growth. Moreover, throughout the life of the human or animal being, within many tissues, they act as a reserve of cells for repair processes, with the almost unlimited ability to replicate and to replace other damaged or dead cells. When a stem cell divides, each new cell originating from it has the potential both to remain an identical cell to the initial one (self-reproduction) and to specialize in any other type of cell with a specific function (specialization), such as a muscle, bone, cartilage, blood or nervous system cell.

The main categories of stem cells are embryonic, perinatal tissue cells, and adult (or somatic) cells. In 1981, stem cells from an animal embryo were isolated for the first time. In 1998 James Thomson, University of Madison, Wisconsin, isolated the first line of human embryonic stem cells. These were undifferentiated cells capable of giving rise to 210 different types of cells, representative of the tissues contained in the human body. Stem cells obtained from the embryo are totipotent cells, that is, capable of generating all types of cells. Their use, however, has complex ethical implications because their extraction can cause damage to the embryo. Perinatal stem cells, such as those of the umbilical cord and adult non-stem cells, instead involving particular ethical problems, are in the already formed human organism and have multipotency characteristics, that is, able to produce different types of specialized cells of the body, but not all types. These cells have the function of increasing the organism and generating new cells for the maintenance and repair of its organs and tissues, thanks to the ability to specialize in certain types of cells. The discovery of stem cells in the umbilical cord dates back to 1978. A significant amount of stem cells can be extracted from the latter through a safe and painless sampling. Procedures for taking adult stem cells from a person allow the collection of fewer cells and are often invasive, causing a certain degree of pain to the individual. Mesenchymal stem cells (MSCs) are an example of adult stem cells. They can self-renew and differentiate in vitro into cells of the mesodermal line, such as chondrocytes, bone cells (osteoblasts), and fat cells (adipocytes). Some studies suggest that mesenchymal stem cells may be able to differentiate even into cell types that do not relate to the mesoderm, such as nerve cells, heart muscle cells, liver cells, and endothelial cells that form the innermost layer of blood vessels. In addition, MSCs have the ability to produce bioactive molecules. They are strong inhibitors of the pro-inflammatory process by stimulating anti-inflammatory mechanisms useful for the regeneration and restorative treatment of tissues and inflammatory diseases. Therefore, it is of particular importance to turn attention to the study of the isolation, manipulation, and multiplication of MSCs because each of these steps can influence their characteristics and, consequently, the result of their action.

Origin and role

Despite multiple pre-clinical and clinical studies, the origin of mesenchymal stem cells and their role in tissue repair have long remained elusive. In 1923 Zimmerman coined the word "pericytes" to indicate those cells that adhere to the outer part of the capillaries, around which extend long ramifications, also called "wall cells."Pericytes have very close contact with endothelial cells. They share the basement membrane in capillaries, arterioles, and venules; they play a fundamental role in angiogenesis, physically stabilize the microvascular network and regulate blood pressure in the microvasculature. In recent years, moreover, it has been discovered that pericytes and other perivascular cells possess tissue regeneration properties. Crisan and collaborators, driven by observations regarding the molecular similarities between pericytes and MSCs, isolated pericytes from different pre- and post-natal human tissues by flow cytofluorimetry and found cultured pericytes are virtually indistinguishable from conventionally in vitro cultured MSCs [1]. In particular, in the presence of appropriate stimuli, cultured pericytes demonstrate the typical ability of mesenchymal stem cells to differentiate into bone, cartilage, fat, and skeletal muscle cells. The same group also identified another population of perivascular cells, located at the level of the adventitious tunic that surrounds the arteries and veins, endowed with the same potential to give rise to authentic MSCs in culture [2]. The perivascular space has, therefore, assumed a role of widespread "niche" of cells endowed with remarkable plasticity during development and regenerative potential. The set of studies in recent years has shown that MSCs are mesodermal progenitors that can be isolated from all vascularized tissues. They play a fundamental role in homeostasis/cell renewal during development and repair following activation by cell damage. Therefore, many argue that mesenchymal stem cells and pericytes are the same cellular entity.

The reparative capacity of MSCs has resulted in their extensive study and use for tissue engineering and regenerative medicine applications since the early 90s in order to reconstruct damaged or degenerated tissues. Recent research has helped to understand better the mechanism of action of these cells once implanted, especially since in some experimental contexts, tissue repair has been obtained in an area distant from the implantation site, so it has been deduced that tissue healing can be achieved through the secretion of growth factors, the production of extracellular vesicles and the interaction with the immune system by MSCs. An evolution of the concept of MSCs from the "brick" of tissue engineering to the concept of "conductor" of the cellular repair mechanism has therefore taken place. In particular, extracellular vesicles derived from MSCs and their therapeutic potential are currently the subject of numerous studies to support indirect use by these cells with a "cell-free" system [3]. Extracellular vesicles are particles derived from cells surrounded by a membrane that acts as spacecraft carrying a wide range of biomolecules to different target cells. They play a crucial role in maintaining cellular homeostasis and different processes, both physiological and pathological. They, therefore, have an important diagnostic and therapeutic significance and have been studied in different fields, both in vitro and in vivo. Mesenchymal stem cells have also been extensively studied as prolific producers of extracellular vesicles. The latter has been examined as a therapeutic alternative to MSCs themselves as they potentially have similar therapeutic effects but constitute a "cell-free" system. Extracellular vesicles derived from MSCs have been studied for regenerative medicine and tissue engineering applications. More importantly, it has several advantages over the use of cells, such as lower immunogenicity and the ability to cross biological barriers, and fewer safety concerns.

Mesenchymal stem cells play a specific role in all three stages of tissue repair. In the first phase, the MSCs are induced to migrate to the damaged tissue from the nearest niche thanks to the action of the cytokines released by the damaged tissue itself and arrived on site begin to secrete in turn cytokines that serve to conclude the phase of inflammation of the tissue. During the second phase of repair, the cells of the damaged tissue must not suffer further damage and begin to proliferate in order to replace the cells that have died as a result of the insult. In this phase, which generally lasts a couple of weeks, MSCs secrete a number of anti-apoptotic and proliferation-inducing factors to stimulate the mitosis of damaged tissue cells. In the third phase, which can last several months, MSCs secrete angiogenic factors that underlie the

neo-vascularization of tissue in order to promote the final stage of remodeling and maturation.
Regenerative medicine is a field applicable in various specialties. This evolving field is taking over most traditional therapies. It combines stem cells, biomaterials, and growth factors to repair damaged organs or tissues by relying on rapid and efficient tissue growth. Regenerative medicine is based on two different pillars. The first concerns cell therapy, and the second is tissue engineering. A cell suspension is injected directly into the damaged tissue in cell therapy. This technique is used to repair tissues to regain their function. However, this approach is generally not sufficient to repair significant tissue defects. An alternative approach is tissue engineering, i.e., the use of cells, generally expanded, associated with biomaterials suitable for the defect and the tissue to be repaired. Such an approach is more complex for problems due to the logistics of cell expansion, vascularization, and the biocompatibility characteristics of the materials themselves.
As we have mentioned, several sources of mesenchymal stem cells can be used in the clinical setting. It is essential to consider that from several studies in the literature, it has emerged that the source from which the stem cell derives determines different peculiarities. In particular, the effectiveness of the differentiation capacity to replace or restore the function of damaged tissues or organs is different. Therefore, choosing the proper stem cell source is critical to achieving positive results in regenerative medicine.

Mesenchymal stem cells sources: practical considerations

Historically, mesenchymal stem cells have been isolated from the bone marrow, and only subsequently other alternative sources have been identified in both perinatal (fig.1) and adult (fig.2) tissues. The MSCs obtained from the various sources have many characteristics that unite them and few distinct peculiarities, such as the expression of some surface markers or the greater propensity to differentiate in vitro towards a given lineage. For example, it is generally recognized that MSCs isolated from bone marrow have more remarkable ability to differentiate towards osteogenic lineage than those isolated from adipose tissue.

The fact that there are so many potential sources of mesenchymal stem cells to be used for therapeutic purposes is a huge advantage because it leaves certain freedom of choice in planning a clinical development of the use of these cells in order to meet both the

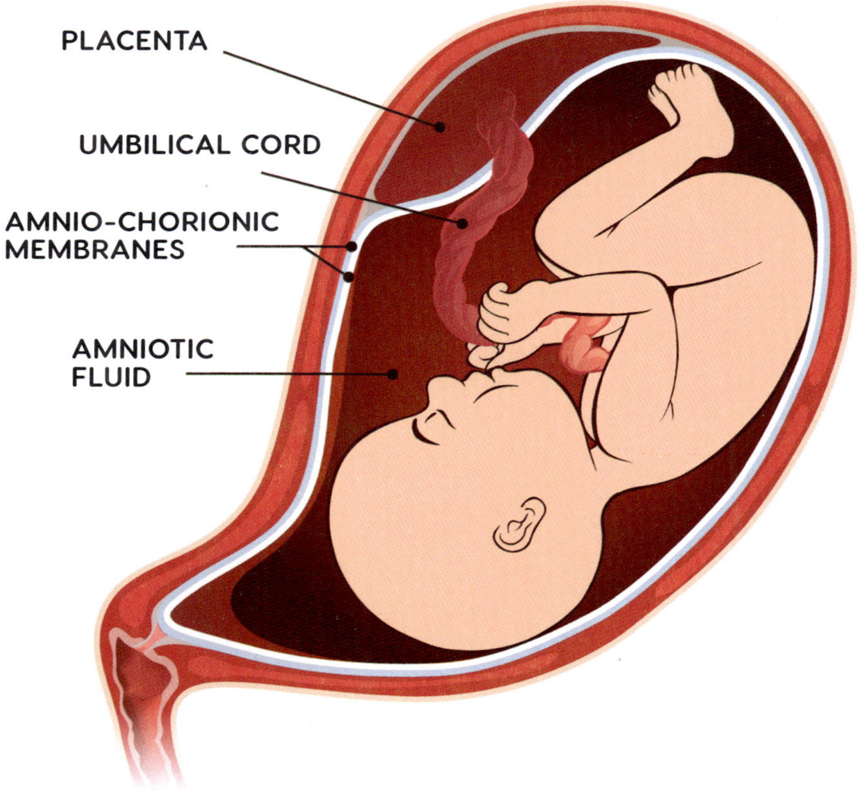

Figure 1 Perinatal tissues

technical needs of the study and the organizational ones of the isolation protocol and possible expansion of the cells. Every potential mesenchymal stem cells source has advantages and limitations. For example, MSCs derived from perinatal tissues are obtained without the recipient having to undergo a sample, and this, in addition to having an advantage in terms of pain for the patient, reduces the procedure to implantation alone: mesenchymal stem cells can be isolated in advance and expanded in time planning the necessary time interval. Although this last aspect seems of little relevance, it has a great impact. Given that MSCs from perinatal

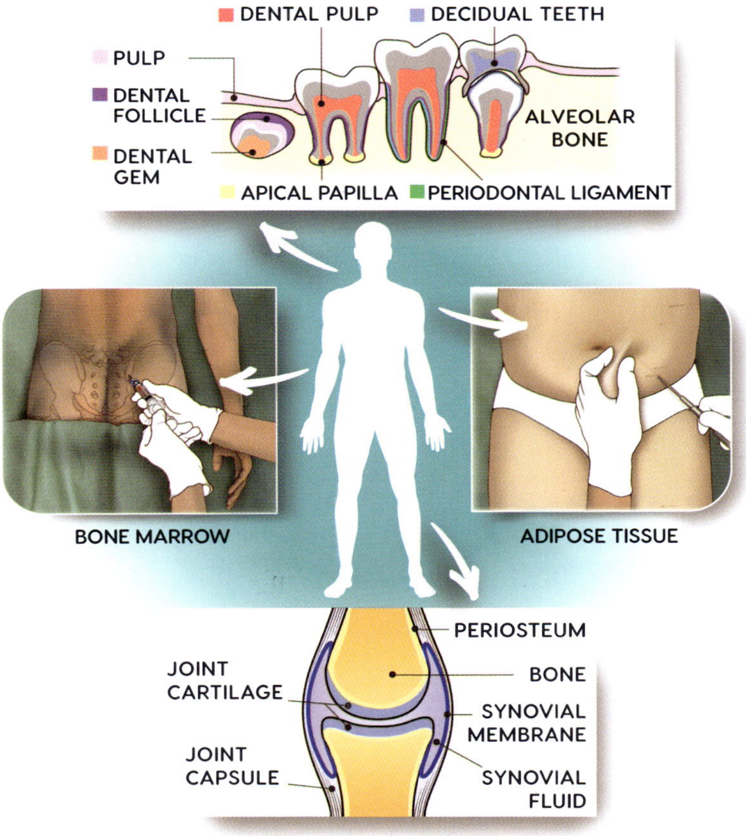

Figure 2 Adult tissues

tissues can be isolated and expanded preventively, these cells can be used for pathologies according to planning. The implant must be done immediately after the damage. However, the availability of cells of perinatal origin is limited because, in Western societies, the number of births has significantly reduced over the years. Therefore, the number of donors for this type of cells is modest. This is especially true when compared to the potential number of donors of adult tissue, such as fat, which is potentially always available in most adults and can be taken more than once. It should also be considered that the use of cells from perinatal tissues is rarely for autologous use, which implies that a number of specific considerations must be made for this use.

Perinatal MSCs

The amniotic membrane and placenta have been used since the 1940s as a graft to repair wounds in dermatology and ophthalmology. Today, many products are based on these membranes commercially available for use in these fields. These membranes are also used as a source of cells for clinical applications, as we will see in detail for each of them below. These cell sources have the advantage of not having ethical implications because they can be obtained without invasive procedures for the donor and are generally waste tissue. Cells isolated from these membranes are derived from tissues with an early embryological origin and have a higher potential for differentiation than cells derived from postnatal tissues. Another peculiar feature of these cells is that their implantation does not cause an immune response of the recipient. The clinical potential of these cells is based on their paracrine effect through an interaction with the cells of the immune system. For a broad review of clinical trials in which these cells were used, see [4].

Placental-derived MSCs

The placenta is a tissue that has unique characteristics as it is an organ that includes the maternal deciduous and fetal tissue. It is an organ that connects the fetus to the uterine membrane through the umbilical cord. In the placenta, various regions contain cells with stem potential, such as amniotic epithelial cells, amniotic mesenchymal cells, mesenchymal chorion cells, mesenchymal chorion, and trophoblast cells, chorionic villus cells, maternal basal deciduous cells, and cord cells, both cord blood and Wharton jelly.

The placenta has a considerable number of mesenchymal stem cells that play a critical role in the recruitment of cells during vasculogenesis and in the development of the placenta itself. These cells are isolated from the placenta after enzymatic digestion removes the umbilical cord and outer membranes. Mesenchymal stem cells obtained from the placenta have been shown to have a proliferative capacity much higher than those derived from other perinatal tissues or bone marrow. They also express cytokeratin, which is quite rare in adult tissue mesenchymal stem cells.

MSCs derived from the amniotic membrane

Mesenchymal stem cells can be isolated from the amniotic membrane after mechanical dissociation of the same from the chorion membrane. In particular, the outer layer of the amniotic membrane that is close to the chorion is particularly rich in stem cells. Studies have shown that amniotic membrane cells have an anti-inflammatory action because they act broadly on the immune system cells, suppress the proliferation of activated T cells, act on B lymphocytes, and block the differentiation of monocytes dendritic cells.

MSCs derived from amniotic fluid

Mesenchymal stem cells obtained from amniotic fluid can be isolated by a fluid sampling during an amniocentesis between the 14th and 16th week of pregnancy or during cesarean delivery. Within the amniotic fluid, there are three adherent cells: an epithelioid population consisting of cuboidal cells derived from the fetal endothelium, a fibroblastoid population generated by fibrous tissue, and the mesenchymal stem cells deriving from the fetal membrane. A characteristic feature of these cells is that they are more "immunoprivilegiate" than MSCs derived from other tissues.

MSCs derived from the chorionic membrane

The chorionic membrane contains both the trophoblastic cells of the chorion and the MSCs. The latter is derived from the reticular layer of the chorion. Once the chorion membrane is mechanically separated from the amniotic membrane, it is dissociated into small pieces of membrane, and following enzymatic digestion with collagenase, the MSCs are isolated. Given the fetal origin of these cells, one of their peculiarities is a high multipotentiality compared to other MSCs.

MSCs derived from chorionic villi

The chorionic villi constitute the embryonic part of the placenta, are rich in capillaries, and allow the regulation of gas exchanges, nourishment, and waste substances between mother and fetus. Chorionic villus sampling consists of aspiration of a small amount of chorionic tissue (30-40 mg) and has been done over a long period of time as a prenatal diagnosis technique. However, the number of cells that can be isolated from chorionic villi is limited because the tissue that can be taken is small in size. Usually, from 40 mg of tissue, you can get between 10,000 and 20,000 cells. Given the small number of cells that can be obtained, this source is more useful for studies on the biology of these cells than for therapeutic uses.

Umbilical cord-derived MSCs

The umbilical cord contains two arteries and a vein surrounded by Wharton jelly. The mesenchymal stem cells deriving from the umbilical cord tissue are obtained by enzymatic digestion of the tissue composed mainly of proteoglycans and hyaluronic acid and have a peculiarity compared to those taken from the umbilical cord blood. If transplanted, they do not need compatibility. The umbilical cord is an interesting source of MSCs that has two advantages: the easy withdrawal of cells as it is a tissue that is often accepted for therapeutic use by cord banks, and the fact that these cells retain some early stem cell genes and, therefore if and when they are expanded in the laboratory they multiply much faster compared to those taken from other sources. Umbilical cord tissue is, therefore, a very rich source of MSC, and the collection of these cells is completely non-invasive.

MSCs from adult fabric

Adult MSCs are present in many tissues of our body and have the great advantage of being able to be taken and implanted in the same patient, greatly reducing the potential risk of transmission of diseases from individual to individual. In addition to autologous use, these cells have the advantage of always being present in the donor. Therefore there is no need to store them in a bank even if numerous studies show that the quality of MSCs in the various tissues of our body would worsen with time. In turn, the tissues change with age. For example, the amount of fat present in the bone marrow increases with age and is present in a high percentage in the elderly. Scientific studies have found that mesenchymal stem cells taken from adipose tissue are less prone to aging than bone marrow. It should also be considered that the onset of certain pathologies in the elderly, the intake of drugs, and the change of lifestyle, could be factors that modify, if not prejudice, the withdrawal of MSCs from some sources.

Bone marrow derived MSCs

The bone marrow source was the first source of stem cells. Bone marrow aspirate has been used for more than 50 years to obtain hematopoietic stem cells in transplants for hematological diseases. In the bone marrow cavity reside different cell populations, including mesenchymal stem cells that perform different functions, including the maintenance of the hematopoietic stem cells themselves, and possess interesting characteristics of plasticity and transdifferentiation. Bone marrow harvesting is an invasive and potentially painful procedure, so it is generally done under general anesthesia. Usually, a suction of 50 ml of bone marrow blood is performed, which is then concentrated by means of systems that usually employ the centrifugation of the total marrow to obtain a concentrate of mononucleated cells. This bone marrow concentrate, in which the mesenchymal stem cells content is then enriched, can be used as such at therapeutic level, or the cells can proceed to a selective expansion of the MSCs in vitro. Bone marrow as a source of mesenchymal stem cells has been the most common source because initially the mesenchymal stem cells were used for applications in the musculoskeletal field, and technically, the removal of marrow is a standard procedure in the orthopedic field. At the same time, doctors specialized in other disciplines may find the procedure complex and impractical. Although bone marrow remains the most widely recognized source of MSCs for clinical use, due to the painful and invasive procedure for its collection, other MSCs sources have aroused the scientific community's interest.

MSCs derived from periosteum

The periosteum is a thin, richly vascularized membrane that covers the outer surface of the bone. The osteogenic property of the periosteum has been known for many centuries because it is used clinically to induce fracture repair. The periosteum has isolated mesenchymal stem cells since the early 90s of the last century. As a source of MSCs, it is easy to obtain it for research purposes because it can be taken from bone tissue discarded in the surgical room during elective surgeries, such as hip replacement. It is more difficult to use it as a source of mesenchymal stem cells for clinical use because the sampling requires specific surgery that leaves an area of morbidity in the patient. The amount of tissue that can be obtained is relatively modest.

MSCs derived from adipose tissue

Adipose tissue is an excellent source of mesenchymal stem cells because it is easy to access and widely available, being a tissue present in most of the world population.

Cells from subcutaneous adipose tissue

The subcutaneous adipose tissue has a complexity and a dynamism that, even today, we have not fully understood. In all likelihood, the interest in adipose tissue as a source of mesenchymal stem cells has led to studying this tissue in more depth and understanding some aspects that had not been described until now. To cite an example, an interesting study [5] has shown that the type of cells that can be isolated from fat is different in a female population under the age of 35 compared to that of a female population over 45 years, concluding that adipose tissue undergoes a radical change over the years in its cellular composition.

Adipose tissue is defined as the best source because the percentage of mesenchymal stem cells in the taken tissue corresponds to 1%, against 0.01% of the bone marrow. It is a complex tissue formed by different cell types: preadipocytes, mature adipocytes, smooth muscle cells, fibroblasts, monocytes, endothelial cells, macrophages, lymphocytes, and mesenchymal cells. Adipose tissue can be obtained through a biopsy or liposuction, with the advantage of a less invasive sampling and therefore associated with less morbidity than mesenchymal stem cells obtained from bone marrow. After being taken and reduced to minimal pieces, the tissue is subjected to enzymatic digestion by the enzyme collagenase type II. After digestion and centrifugation, the pellet that remains is concentrated of various cell populations and is referred to as Stromal vascular fraction (SVF). The cells obtained in SVF can be cultured to be expanded, and once a homogeneous culture of adherent cells is obtained, these are defined as Adipose-derived stem cells (ASCs). Adipose tissue is usually accumulated in the abdomen, hips, thighs, buttocks, or arms. Depending on the anatomical region from which it is taken, the mesenchymal stem cells isolated from it may have different densities and characteristics. For example, arm fat has the highest concentration of MSCs.

MSCs derived from the Bichat Bubble

This adipose tissue is contained within the cheeks between the masseter muscle and the buccinator muscle. Since 1977 the transplantation or removal of this tissue has been used to correct congenital alterations of the oral or oronasal cavity. This tissue is removed and discarded frequently by plastic surgeons to reduce the cheeks volume in obese people. Since an incision can easily take it in the inner part of the cheek without leaving scars, this tissue is a source of mesenchymal stem cells of choice for those who want to use MSCs in reconstruction applications in oral and maxillofacial surgery.

MSCs derived from Hoffa's wad

Hoffa's wad is a pad of adipose tissue placed in the knee under the patella, between the patellar tendon, the femoral condyle, and the tibial plate. It is an intracapsular structure, but it is outside the synovium. Due to its location, it can be an easy-to-access source of mesenchymal stem cells during knee surgery. In addition, during a knee prosthesis surgery, Hoffa's wad is generally waste material, so it is easy to obtain samples of it to study it. As adipose tissue, it has a concentration of cells and, in particular, of mesenchymal stem cells, much higher than subcutaneous fat.

MSCs derived from the synovial membrane

The synovial membrane is a component of the synovium in direct contact with the fibrous membrane on the outer surface and with the synovial fluid on the inner surface. The internal one that communicates with the joint cavity has no blood vessels, while the external one is rich. Mesenchymal cells derived from the synovium have a high proliferative capacity, are poorly immunogenic, and have a high ability to differentiate towards the cartilaginous line. Synovial membrane mesenchymal stem cells are generally chosen in cartilage regeneration applications for all these reasons.

MSCs derived from the endometrium

The endometrium is a tissue that regenerates regularly. The endometrium has three cell populations: epithelial progenitor cells, endothelial progenitor cells, and mesenchymal stem cells. mesenchymal stem cells can be isolated by tissue biopsies or by menstrual blood collection. These cells have characteristics very similar to the MSCs of other tissues. If collected from menstrual blood, their collection is not invasive nor painful. The fact remains that women of childbearing age can only obtain these cells, so in an autologous implant area, only part of the world population can be a candidate. On the other hand, it is certainly an advantage that these cells can be obtained approximately 400 times over the fertile life.

MSCs derived from the orofacial area

Cells derived from the orofacial area include all cells isolated from different sites in the oral cavity. These cells have been the subject of many studies in the dental field, primarily because those who work in this sector mainly perform surgeries limited to the oral cavity carried out in surgical rooms that are not within a classic hospital context, so for a professional in the sector it is not easy to be able to perform a sample from the iliac crest, or adipose tissue of the patient. The cells of the tissues of the orofacial area have peculiarities that are often derived from the influence of the microenvironment in which these cells grow.

There are eight cell populations derived from the orofacial area that include:

- MSCs derived from the dental pulp. The dental pulp is a connective tissue of mesenchymal origin, vascularized and rich in nerve endings that develops from the dental papilla. The tissue is located in the innermost part of the tooth. It is surrounded by enamel and dentin, excluding apart at the base of the roots where a hole allows the passage of a blood vessel, a lymphatic vessel, and a nerve. The MSCs obtained from the dental pulp were the first to be isolated and characterized in this area, mainly because they can be isolated from the teeth removed without invasive procedures for the patient. Thanks to their multipotentiality, this type of cell has been widely used for preclinical research in regenerative medicine, especially for validating biomaterials.

- MSCs derived from decidual teeth. These cells are easy to obtain because they derive from milk teeth that are replaced by permanent teeth in a certain period of growth. They are the subject of high interest because they have many characteristics of immature cells. The limitation of this cell source derives from the fact that the change of the dentition occurs only once in the life of an individual and that the prediction of the tooth does not always take place in a mode or a temporal context compatible with the collection of cells.
- MSCs derived from periodontal ligament. The periodontal ligament is a connective structure that loosens the root cement to the alveolar bone and has a fundamental function in keeping the tooth inside the bone, allowing it to cushion the chewing loads of the tooth. This tissue contains a population of cells that has the task of maintaining and regenerating the tissue itself. Many studies have shown that mesenchymal stem cells derived from the periodontal ligament have a high clonogenicity and differentiate, especially towards the osteogenic line. For these reasons, it constitutes a potential source of MSCs for bone tissue reconstruction in dental applications.
- MSCs derived from the dental follicle. The dental follicle is a tissue that envelops and protects the dental bud. Its primary function is to regulate the dental rash, and it is

a progenitor of the periodontium, which is the apparatus that constitutes the attachment of the teeth. To obtain mesenchymal stem cells from this tissue, it is necessary to isolate them from the tooth follicle at the beginning of root formation. The dental follicle can be obtained from wisdom teeth even in adulthood. In particular, these cells have a strong immunomodulatory capacity and have been successfully used in patients with Crohn's disease to reduce inflammation.

- MSCs derived from alveolar bone. The alveolar bone is the bone that surrounds the dental alveoli, which forms the basis of attachment of the teeth. The alveolar bone is perforated by the apical foramen that allows the passage of vessels and nerves to the teeth. Since 2009, mesenchymal stem cells have been isolated from this tissue and used in preclinical studies. Access to the hive bone is not difficult because it is sufficient to move the gum. However, the amount of alveolar bone taken without creating excessive damage is limited.
- MSCs derived from the apical papilla.The apical papilla is a soft tissue present during the development of permanent teeth at their apex. This tissue has the function of helping the formation of teeth and later will become the dental pulp. From this, it follows that this tissue can only be obtained at certain stages of the development of permanent teeth. Mesenchymal stem cells can be isolated either by enzymatic digestion or spontaneously, as cells can independently migrate from the tissue to the culture plate.
- MSCs derived from the dental gem. This type of cell is isolated from the dental bud of the included third molar. A peculiarity of the mesenchymal stem cells derived from the dental bud is that they have a proliferative capacity higher than other types of cells isolated from adult tissues: these cells have been kept in culture for at least 60 duplications in a brief time.
- Gum-derived MSCs. The gum is a scaly epithelial tissue with a blade

of connective tissue attached to the bone tissue on one side and covered with a keratinized epithelium that ensures its functions within the biological barrier oral cavity. It is an easy-to-access mesenchymal stem cells source during a normal oral surgery session and has the unique feature of regenerating without leaving scar tissue. The mesenchymal stem cells isolated from the gum have been used for reconstruction interventions in the musculoskeletal and dermatological fields. Moreover, thanks to their immunomodulating action, they have also been used in oncology [6].

MSCs of animal origin

Alexander Friedenstein first isolated the mesenchymal stem cells in 1976 from the bone marrow of a guinea pig. Therefore, it was confirmed that mesenchymal stem cells could be isolated from tissues of animal origin before the finding.

MSCs could also be obtained from the human marrow. Currently, mesenchymal stem cells are isolated from tissues of many animal species, not only from mammals. They are used, as well as for research purposes, as therapeutic agents to treat various diseases in the veterinary field, both in utility animals and in those of affection. Whether the mesenchymal stem cells obtained from animals is comparable to those of human origin is a question that has not yet been answered. Morphologically, the mesenchymal stem cells of animal origin are similar to the human ones. There is also a certain correspondence of the surface proteins expressed by these types of cells.

On the other hand, the proliferation of cells of animal origin is generally higher than that of human cells. It is difficult to understand whether this higher mitotic index of cells of animal origin is due to the intrinsic characteristics of the cells themselves or because the means and conditions of culture used to cultivate MSCs are not yet optimal for human cells. In contrast, they are optimal for animal ones.

Another important consideration concerns the homology of the tissues from which animal mesenchymal stem cells are taken compared to the human tissue. However, as far as bone marrow is concerned, there is a macroscopic similarity between the human marrow and most mammals in relation to function and cell populations. If we analyze adipose tissue, we can see that its distribution and composition are very different from species to species. Mammals, especially small ones, or hibernating ones, have a higher brown fat component than humans have, where brown fat tissue is present only in small amounts that become active when the body is exposed to very low temperatures. So, while we know that mesenchymal stem cells can be isolated from the fat of many animals, we cannot be sure that the cells are homologous to the human ones being the starting tissue different. A real comparative research would be necessary to be sure of any similarities and differences between cells of human and animal origin.

The issue of homology between animal and human mesenchymal stem cells has profound implications because it impacts the development of animal models necessary to validate the safety and therapeutic efficacy of expanded MSCs in vitro. The expanded mesenchymal stem cells must be considered a drug for the European legislation. Therefore, the MSC expansion must follow the good manufacturing practice (GMP) guidelines. The drug's effectiveness is demonstrated following the guidelines of good clinical practice (Good Clinical Practice, GCP). Therefore, it is essential to understand whether the results obtained in preclinical animal models are also applicable to humans. To give an example: if an ovine model is used to demonstrate that expanded mesenchymal stem cells sown on a material can be effective for the reconstruction of a cartilage defect and expanded mesenchymal stem cells of sheep origin are used, the question that must be asked is: the drug (i.e., sheep expanded MSCs) that I use in the experimental model is equivalent to what I would use in humans (i.e., human expanded mesenchymal stem cells)? Only if the answer is yes, the results obtained in animal testing can be used as preclinical validation of the drug's effectiveness for a clinical trial. Otherwise, they can only be used for veterinary practice.

In conclusion, the evidence that mesenchymal stem cells are present in many animal species indicates that these cells perform an essential physiological function and have a potential therapeutic utility that has been highly preserved during the evolution of animal species. How much animal mesenchymal stem cells are representative of human ones is an aspect that needs more study, and that should be a strand of interest that is desirable to be the subject of further research.

Conclusions

Mesenchymal stem cells can be isolated from different tissues implying an almost unlimited number of opportunities. The optimal source of MSCs for applications in regenerative medicine must be made after considering many aspects such as the practicality of the collection and implantation in terms of organization, the characteristics of the cells, and the number of cells I want to implant. A very important aspect not to be underestimated is also to make specific considerations in the design of preclinical studies to ensure that the mesenchymal stem cells used in the animal model are homologous to those used in the clinical study.

References

1. Crisan M, Yap S, Casteilla L, Chen WC, Corselli M, Park TS et al. A perivascular origin for mesenchymal stem cells in multiple human organs. Cell Stem Cell 3:301 (2008).
2. Corselli M, Chen CW, Sun B, Yap S, Rubin JP, Péault B. The tunica adventitia of human arteries and veins as a source of mesenchymal stem cells. Stem Cells Dev 21:1299 (2012).
3. Zhao AG, Shah K, Cromer B, Sumer H. Mesenchymal Stem Cell-Derived Extracellular Vesicles and Their Therapeutic Potential. Stem Cells Int. PMID: 32908543 (2020 Aug)
4. Silini AE, Cargnoni A, Magatti M, Pianta

S, Parolini O. The long path of human placenta, and its derivatives, in regenerative medicine. Frontiers in Bionegineering and Biotechnology 3: 162 (2015)

5. De Girolamo L, Lopa S, Arrigoni E, Sartori MF, Baruffaldi Preis FW, Brini AT. Human adipose-derived stem cells isolated from young and elderly women: their differentiation potential and scaffold interaction during in vitro osteoblastic differentiation. Cytotherapy 11: 793 (2009)
6. Zhang QZ, Nguyen AL, Yu WH, Le AD. Human Oral Mucosa and Gingiva. J Dent Res 91:1011 (2012)

CHAPTER 10

REGENERATIVE THERAPY OF THE MUSCULOSKELETAL SYSTEM: THE SCAFFOLDS

Giuseppe M. Peretti[1,2], Michele Lombardo[3], Laura Mangiavini[1,2]

1) IRCCS Galeazzi Orthopaedic Institute, Milan, Italy

2) Department of Biomedical Sciences for Health, University of Milan, Milan, Italy

3) Residency Program in Orthopedics and Traumatology, University of Milan, Milan, Italy

Introduction

Scaffolds in the orthopedic field represent a significant innovation to optimize tissue reparative and regenerative strategies.

Scaffolds are biomaterials used as scaffolding for cells that create the most favorable environment for their proliferation and growth to generate an "engineered tissue." The ultimate goal of developing an engineered tissue is to treat the loss of substance and function of the various target organs or tissues. Scaffolds are undoubtedly the co-protagonist, along with cells, for engineered tissue formation.

The development of an engineered tissue requires different professional figures with different skills. To get to the clinical application of engineered tissue, it is necessary to follow a transversal path that starts from materials science and cell biology, to move on to biochemistry and molecular biology to, ultimately, arrive at surgical practice [1].

There are different ways to engineer tissues. Most commonly used are "*in vitro*" and "*in vivo*."

The "in vitro" model consists of the production in the laboratory of vital tissue and its consequent implantation at the patient's recipient site. Undoubted advantages of this technique are the possibility of studying the structure of the fabric before its implantation [2]. With the "in vivo" technique, the scaffold is instead implanted without cells in the donor site, and here the process of development of the new tissue will begin. It will then be populated by the target cells that will begin matrix synthesis and then the formation of the tissue itself: the patient is used as an incubation chamber and bioreactor for tissue regeneration.

The scaffold must possess a series of physical and chemical characteristics. It must first be biocompatible to not trigger reactions of rejection, intolerance, or allergies in the host. It must be bio-integrated: materials implanted in patients' bodies, such as joint or vascular prostheses, are biocompatible but will never be populated by a cell population of the host. A scaffold must have specific mechanical properties: think of the stresses it must withstand if positioned in certain districts, such as in the loading areas of the joints of the lower limbs. The structural architecture, such as porosity characteristics, is also fundamental to maximize the possibilities in terms of colonization of a specific cell population and bio integration.

The biomaterials currently available to us are polymers, natural or synthetic, or ceramics.

Ceramics have a high structural rigidity at the cost of deficient elasticity. They possess an intricate and fragile surface and are widely used for bone and osteochondral defects, such as hydroxyapatite.

Among the disadvantages of this type of biomaterial, we must include the fragility, the difficulty of modeling, and the slow degradation time.

Natural polymers are biologically active and promote cell migration and engraftment. They are biodegradable and favor host cells for the production of extracellular matrix, which progressively replaces polymers as they undergo degradation and resorption; however, they have very few mechanical properties and their reproducibility in terms of characteristics still represents a challenge.

Synthetic polymers can be manufactured with specific three-dimensional structures, and their degradation rate can be varied, changing the chemical composition of the scaffold itself. However, their biointegration is more complex and their reduced bioactivity; there is a risk of tissue rejection, and they can cause necrosis as they are often associated with a low pH.

The future of biomaterials is represented by composite biomaterials, which arise from the union of different types of biomaterials to mimic as faithfully as possible the tissue architecture you want to develop. These may also have bio-instructive characteristics. They will instruct colonizing cells on how to differentiate and what matrix to produce through stimuli inherent in the scaffold itself, such as growth factors, bioactive peptides, and cytokines. They can also be used as vehicles of therapeutic genes, thus defining a new concept of gene therapy. Modulating the mechanical properties of the scaffold, it will be possible to condition the variations of mechano-transduction and the consequent cellular behavior.

We will now proceed with the analysis of the scaffolds and biomaterials used in common orthopedic practice and those of more recent experimentation.

Cartilage

The use of scaffolds for cartilage arises from the need to cover areas of substance loss, more or less large and more or less localized [3].

There is a plethora of biomaterials used in common clinical practice, but before we go into their description, we need to distinguish between cartilage lesions. They can be pure chondral lesions, where articular cartilage is lost, or osteochondral lesions, where cartilage loss is also added to subchondral bone damage [4].

For chondral lesions, so-called *one-step* procedures can be performed, where surgery is performed in a single session. We can have transplants of cartilaginous fragments, application of scaffolds without cells, preceded or not by tissue activation [5].

One of the first techniques used was the one that involved the use of a flap of periosteum to cover the cartilage defect, but having the foresight to make a rotation of 180 ° to the flap, so that the cambial layer of the periosteum was facing the center of the articular cavity.

Another technique involves the affixing of a membrane at the level of the site of loss of substance, after bone marrow stimulation, for example, with microfractures; this is the case of the A.M.I.C. technique (*Autologous matrix-induced Chondrogenesis*) where the blood clot is covered and protected with the implantation of a collagen membrane. This implant protects the stem cells and gives the cells themselves the proper stimulus to generate repair cartilage tissue.

For the treatment of cartilage lesions, there may also be so-called *two-step* techniques. There is an intermediate step between the collection and the culture grafting of the cell population of interest.

We must include the A.C.I. technique (*Autologous Chondrocyte Implantation*), which involves cartilage sampling from non-load areas, cell culture, and subsequent reimplantation in the area to be treated followed by a covering of the graft with biological (periosteum) or biocompatible material. The M.A.C.I (*Matrix-induced Autologous Chondrocyte Implantation*) technique differs from the latter because the cultured chondrocytes are sown on a membrane that is directly used as a cover for the cartilage defect.

Innovative therapy, still in the experimental phase (currently in phase II of experimentation), is the so-called nose-to-knee [6]. This is a two-step therapy, which involves the removal of a portion of the nasal septum, the enzymatic digestion of the matrix, and the isolation of nasal chondrocytes, their cell culture, and their subsequent sowing a collagen scaffold. The study currently underway in phase 2 involves two experimental arms: the first in which the cells are seeded on the membrane for only two days; the second in which the cells are sown on the membrane for two weeks (schematizing, one is represented by a carrier matrix immature chondrocytes, the other from engineered cartilage). The second step of the procedure involves the implantation of this biomaterial at the level of the chondral defect.

The preliminary results of this study would seem to envisage the possibility of treating broader defects than classical techniques, lower donor site morbidity, and a higher quality graft.

As for osteochondral defects, the precursor technique was mosaicplasty, which consists of taking osteochondral tablets from areas of non-load of the knee to make full-thickness grafts to fill the defect. Disadvantages of this technique are the morbidity of the donor site and the difficulty or impossibility of a complete filling of the osteochondral defect.

To date, biphasic biomaterials are also used, such as in the Maioregen technique.

These biphasic scaffolds may be cell-less within them or may be seeded by cells.

The future of these techniques will involve the use of gene vectors in order to increasingly precisely target the commitment of the cells seeded on these scaffolds.

Meniscus

As for the scaffolds for meniscal structures, they must have particular characteristics.

They must be biocompatible and biodegradable in the long term. They must be able to allow cellular diffusion and that of nutrients. They must allow the adhesion of growth factors and their controlled release. They must have mechanical properties that withstand the forces transmitted inside the joint and a proper porosity (communication of 150-500 microns). Also, in this case, the scaffolds can be natural or synthetic [7].

The collagen meniscal implant is an example: it comes from the bovine Achilles tendon, which is processed, purified, crosslinked, and freeze-dried. The indications for the use of this implant are pretty stringent: it can only be used for the medial meniscus, which must have an intact meniscal wall, there must be no instability, and can be used for lesions in the red/red area or at most red/white. In addition, it is not indicated for complete meniscal replacements. The results of this technique are not, to date, always entirely satisfactory.

Quite widespread in clinical practice is, to date, the use of PRP (Platelet-Rich Plasma): this is peripheral whole blood that is centrifuged to concentrate platelets: in this case, no type of scaffold is used.

The future of these treatments will involve the implantation of cellular constructs created through specific bioreactors with cells taken from biopsy samples.

Bone

Bone tissue has always been at the center of studies and research, as often, in clinical practice, we often face bone losses, which can be minimal or massive.

Autologous or allogeneic bone grafts have been used for several years to solve this problem. In addition, several bone substitutes have been released on the market, with good osteoconductive properties (they act as a scaffolding for colonization by osteoblasts that will become osteocytes) and osteoinductive (they favor a cellular differentiation towards bone tissue); these can be enriched or not with growth factors, cells or both [8]. Bone substitutes include metals (plates or joint replacement), ceramics (filling of substance losses), and polymers (pure scaffolds or carrying active molecules).

References

1. T. Baudequin and M. Tabrizian, "Multilineage Constructs for Scaffold-Based Tissue Engineering: A Review of Tissue-Specific Challenges," *Advanced Healthcare Materials*. 2018.
2. G.M. Peretti, M. Buragas, C. Scotti, L. Mangiavini, C. Sosio, A. By Giancamillo, C. Domeneghini, G. Fraschini, "An in vitro tissue-engineered model for osteochondral repair," *Sport Sci. Health*, 2006.
3. E. A. Makris, A. H. Gomoll, K. N. Malizos, J.C. Hu, and K. A. Athanasiou, "Repair and tissue engineering techniques for articular cartilage," *Nature Reviews Rheumatology*. 2015.
4. G.M. Peretti, G. Filardo, A. Gigante, L. Mangiavini, A. Marmotti, and M. Ronga, "Pathophysiology of Cartilage Injuries," in *Orthopedic Sports Medicine*, 2011.
5. A. G. Marmotti, G.M. Peretti, S. Mattia, L. Mangiavini, D. E. Bonasia, F. Dettoni, E. Bellato, S. Schwienbacher, F. Castoldi, "One-step cartilage repair with minced chondral fragment onto a composite scaffold: An in vitro human study at low oxygen tension," *J. Biol. Regul. Homeost. Agents*, 2017.
6. M. Mumme, A. Barbero, S. Miot, A.

Wixmerten, S. Feliciano, F. Wolf, A.M. Asnaghi, D. Baumhoer, O. Bieri, M. Kretzschmar, G. Pagenstert,M. Haug, D. J. Schaefer, I. Martin, M. Jakob, "Nasal chondrocyte-based engineered autologous cartilage tissue for repair of articular cartilage defects: an observational first-in-human trial," *Lancet*, 2016.
7. J. Sun, S. Vijayavenkataraman, and H. Liu, "An overview of scaffold design and fabrication technology for engineered knee meniscus," *Materials*. 2017.
8. S. Yin, W. Zhang, Z. Zhang, and X. Jiang, "Recent Advances in Scaffold Design and Material for Vascularized Tissue-Engineered Bone Regeneration," *Advanced Healthcare Materials*. 2019.

CHAPTER 11

BONE MARROW CONCENTRATION SYSTEMS: BONE MARROW ASPIRATE CONCENTRATE (BMAC)

Daniele Pressato[1], Alfredo Franceschini[2]

1) Marketing Manager & Scientific Affairs Novagenit S. r. l.

2) Product Manager Novagenit S.r.l.

Introduction

In the last decade in the orthopedic field, different cellular and biological therapies have established themselves as treatment for musculoskeletal diseases, in particularly for the treatment of degeneration of the joint cartilage and tendons. If we retrace the history of regenerative medicine, we will note that already at the begenning of 2000, orthopedics started to use tissue engineering techniques such as ACI (*Autologous Chondrocyte Implantation*) and MACI (*Matrix-Associated Chondrocyte Implantation*) in the treatment of some degenerative and traumatic diseases affecting articular cartilage [1, 2].

Thus, an evolutionary path was undertaken in the orthopedic field, that was moving from a reparative surgical orientation towards a regenerative approach to stimulate the intrinsic properties of the organism to regenerate connective tissues damaged by trauma or degenerative diseases. It is believed that this process, the result of multidisciplinary research that has combined biomedical sciences, nanotechnologies, and scientific subjects such as the chemistry of biomaterials, has significantly affected orthopedic surgery. Today the terms bio-orthopedics and ortho-biology are at the center of attention and represent, in their respective declinations, and for some categories of patients, an innovative, safe, less invasive therapeutic perspective with proven clinical efficacy and able to provide alternative solutions to traditional surgical treatments.

More recently, among these therapies, the use of autologous bone marrow mesenchymal cells (MSCs) has opened the way to new treatment options for specific pathologies affecting the connective tissues not only of the skeletal system but also of other anatomical regions such as critical ischemia of the lower extremities and ischemic heart disease. However, in the orthopedic field, if the use of the autologous bone marrow concentrate and the devices for obtaining it already represent consolidated practices, the clinical debate has been oriented towards understanding whether or not this practice can be considered a "standard of care" for certain pathological conditions, in particular affecting the articular cartilage or other districts of the skeletal system. Another aspect under discussion is the actual ability of bone marrow concentration devices to provide an adequate number of progenitor cells to be administered to the patient compared to the baseline content, in particular the content of nucleated cells, a cell fraction within which MSCs and growth factors. This debate has generated a further stimulus to research, so much so that new bone marrow sampling systems are appearing on the market that exclude or question the usefulness of the centrifugation process favoring the qualitative cell aspect, supporting an equivalence if not superiority in terms of clinical efficacy compared to the traditional system of bone marrow concentration.

This chapter will investigate some aspects of these technologies and their clinical potential. The results of a systematic review of the literature on the use of concentrated bone marrow aspirate and related processing systems will be described, furthermore, through the creation of new systems that claim to be capable of providing qualitative performance superior to current systems, new technological innovation in this sector is already coming up.

Regenerative medicine in bio-orthopedics

As mentioned, regenerative medicine has entered significantly into the orthopedic surgical specialty to treat specific pathologies such as cartilage lesions or bone lesions that are difficult to heal. Without rule out the need for surgery to restore the correct biomechanics, these methodologies, thanks to a multidisciplinary technological evolution, have proven to represent a safe therapeutic tool for the regeneration of connective tissues, with acceptable clinical results. Evidence shows that young patients with disabling diseases of various kinds can derive critical clinical benefits compared to traditional repair methods [3]. In the treatment of cartilage defects, where surgical approach is not always decisive, it should be emphasized that it allows to postpone the placement of a joint prosthetic implant in most cases.

If we analyze some recent market data, we observe how in the United States, the cell therapies with mesenchymal cells have impressed a significant economic impact. It is estimated that more than 350 companies are marketing systems for cell processing in about 600 health facilities in the country. 61% of companies offer devices to extract stem cells from autologous adipose tissue, while 48% of the market devices (mainly bone marrow concentrators) are for treatments based on cells extracted from autologous bone marrow [4].

The most widespread use of these therapies remains in diseases affecting the musculoskeletal system, with over 300 orthopedic clinics followed by specialized centers for pain therapy, sports medicine, and neurosurgery. To date, the companies that dominate the market are mainly located in North America (54%), Europe (about 20%), China, and the Far East (20%), and the remaining percentage in other countries [5].

The use of autologous bone marrow concentrate, commonly known by the acronym BMAC (*Bone Marrow Aspirate Concentrate*), is one of the most used procedures in orthopedics to amplify the self-repairing regenerative potential of the musculoskeletal system. Looking at the market statistics, in the last 5 years, there has been a steady growth in the number of surgeries where BMAC has been used. In Europe, in the exclusively orthopedic sector, in the period 2015-2019, about 175,000 BMAC implants were carried out with an annual average of 35,000 surgical procedures and an annual growth of more than 7% with corresponding revenues of more than 60 million euros. Short-term projections confirm the positive trend with a forecast of around 200,000 plants for the period 2020-2023, an annual growth of 8%, and revenues of over 65 million euros. It should be considered in any case that the predominant position in the field of regenerative procedures for the treatment of diseases affecting the musculoskeletal system remains in favor of therapy based on Platelet Rich Plasma (PRP), with over 700,000 implants in the period 2015-2019 and a forecast of almost 750,000 applications for the period 2020-2023.

Unlike cell cultures that involve a surgical time of tissue collection, the subsequent culture in the laboratory, and a further intervention for the grafting of the culture, the application of BMAC is a "*one-step*" technique.

The pathologies commonly treated surgically with this technology are chondral and osteochondral defects, avascular necrosis of the femoral epiphysis, bone cysts, pseudoarthrosis, or the treatment at the non-surgical infiltrative level of primary arthrosis of the joints.

In general, MSCs are cells present in the human body. They maintain memory and the ability to differentiate into cells of other connective tissues, therefore, able to guide healing when traumatic or degenerative processes damage these tissues themselves. One of the limitations of this therapeutic approach is represented by the low cellular concentration within the source, in this case, the bone marrow, and this constitutes a determining variable depending on the clinical result.

Bone marrow is a natural source of multipotent adult undifferentiated mesenchymal/stromal cells. According to their differentiation, they have several functions: a hematopoietic function (HSCs – *Hematopoietic Stem Cells*), an angiogenetic/vasculogenetic (EPCs – *Endothelial Progenitor Cells*), a progenitor of the musculoskeletal system (BMSCs - Bone Marrow Stromal Cells). In addition, the bone marrow also contains a significant amount of platelets (PLTs), growth factors, white blood cells, and red blood cells.

However, within the bone marrow, the BMSCs population, a component that is decisive for an excellent clinical *outcome*, is very rarefied (0.001-0.02% of the totality of nucleated cells present) and is strongly dependent on factors such as the age and state of health of the patient [6]. Identify the correlation between the number of nucleated cells, the content of growth factors, and the effectiveness of healing speed of bone, cartilage, and tendon defects, it is important to provide the right concentration of nucleated cells and growth factors during the surgical time [7]. However, it is essential to have tools and technologies capable of providing the maximum concentration of mononuclear cells and excluding other cellular and non-cellular components, lacking a decisive biological function (and, according to some authors, harmful) concerning the process of regeneration of connective tissues [8]. These systems are commonly identified with the commercial term of "bone marrow concentrators" and the final product that is obtained through a gravitational separation or centrifugation, which exploits the different density of the cellular elements and the corpuscular components of the bone marrow blood, is a concentrate consisting of nucleated cells that include monocytes, lymphocytes, hematopoietic mesenchymal cells and mesenchymal stromal cells that together with the platelet fraction and it´s called *buffy coat*.

The BMSCs contained in the concentrated autologous bone marrow aspirate represent the source of precursors most widely used in the orthopedic surgical field. Due to their distinctive characteristics, they represent an ideal cellular source for tissue regeneration: they are obtained from the same patient, they are able to self-renew, they act as immunomodulators by extinguishing inflammation, they can differentiate into different cellular phenotypes (e.g., chondrogenic and osteogenic), they are able to integrate into the connective tissues in which they are transplanted and trigger mainly a regenerative process.

When introduced in the patient, they act through a paracrine mechanism by secreting factors that cause the cells surrounding the recipient tissue to differentiate and become an active part of the healing process by amplifying the regenerative power of the cell therapy itself.

Another important component of

BMAC is the PRP content as a source of growth factors that interact with cells, maintain cell survival, stimulate their proliferation, acting as a joint homeostatic modulating inflammation, and restore a physiological condition.
Based on the pathological picture and surgical evaluation, determined by the type of defect to be repaired and/or the type of regeneration to be stimulated, BMSCs can be used alone or sown on a "matrix" or more commonly "*scaffold*" that can be of autologous origin (of the same patient), homologous (donor tissue)), heterologous (animal), synthetic.
In this chapter, some technical aspects relating to obtaining concentrated bone marrow aspirate have been explored, mainly which technologies and devices are currently available to obtain an optimal yield in terms of cellular content and recovery of BMSCs, a fundamental detail for achieving an acceptable clinical result.
Through a qualitative narrative review rather than a systematic review of the literature, we have provided a general framework to better understand the state of the art of these systems on the market and, in particular, if the therapeutic product obtained from the BMAC can offer guarantees in terms of clinical benefit for the patient.
We have investigated the technological aspect, not entering into the commercial details, with a dive into the future of cell therapies based on MSCs derived from bone marrow.

BMAC and bone marrow concentration systems: literature review

In the literature review, the only search engine consulted was Pubmed, and the following keywords were included: "Bone Marrow Concentrate or (BMC) and Bone Marrow Aspirate Concentrate or (BMAC)" considering the articles (*full-text*) included in the time interval 2000-2020. Guidelines for reporting systematic reviews and Prisma Statement meta-analysis have been used. The inclusion criteria for evaluating the analysis included only clinical studies related to BMAC treatments for musculoskeletal diseases, such as orthopedics, craniomaxillofacial surgery, traumatology. All non-English-language articles, duplicates attributable to the same clinical trial, and all studies related to vascular surgery, neurosurgery of the dental nervous system, and cardiac surgery were excluded.

Data were extracted from the included studies are shown in the "results" section, including the tables. For clinical efficacy, positive results were considered, while the onset of adverse events was evaluated for safety aspects. In addition, negative results, doubtful or inconclusive results were reported (no symptomatic improvement compared to the pre-intervention situation). In the "materials and methods" section, the type of device on the market used for the concentration of the bone marrow aspirate was taken into account with a description of the relative technology. Moreover, with the help of the technical data reported in the commercial data-sheet of each concentration system, a comparison was made between the devices concerning performance (BMAC vs. basal BMA), evaluating the following parameters: concentration of nucleated cells, mononuclear cells, platelets, and cell yield or recovery.

Results: clinical efficacy

The scheme in fig. 1 shows the evaluation criteria of the articles. The research allowed to select (period 2000-2020) 879 publications related to clinical trials resulting from the typed keywords. Considering the inclusion/exclusion criteria and the title of the *abstract*, 124 publications resulting from the same clinical trial (duplicates) were excluded in the first phase. In a second screening, 633 publications relating to surgical applications not linked to the musculoskeletal system were excluded. For the qualitative analysis, 126 articles (*full text* available) were considered, 2 articles were excluded at a later time, for a final number of 124 publications. Considering just the time interval investigated in the research, it is noted

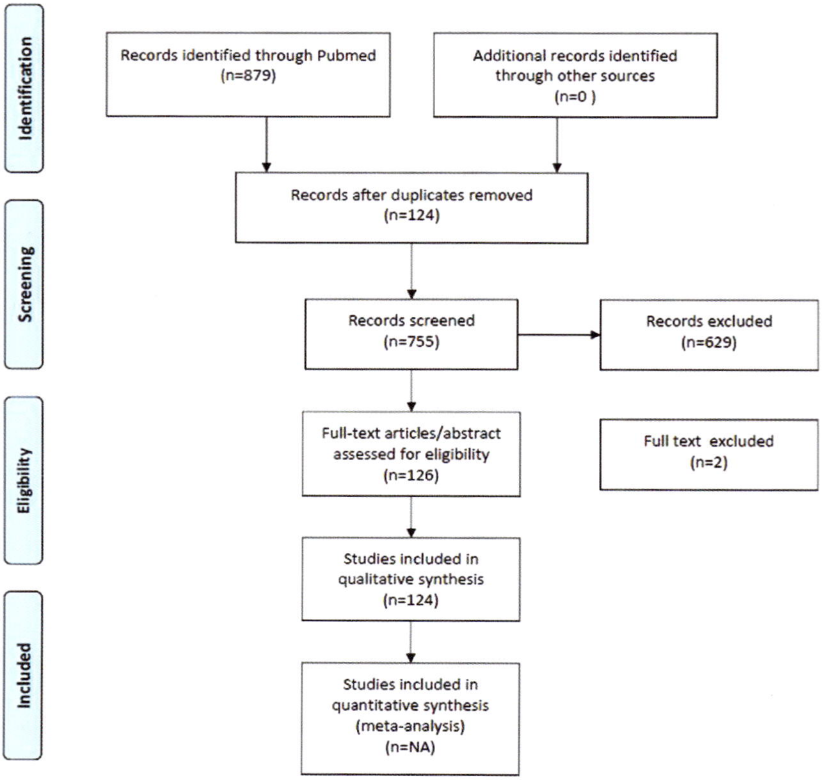

Figure 1 Letter selection criteria according to Prisma statement flow chart

that over the years, in particular in the 2015-2020 range, there has been a significant increase in the number of clinical applications of BMAC (fig. 2). Studies were divided into controlled randomized clinical trials (RCTs), controlled/comparative studies, prospective studies (case series) including case/control, and studies reporting retrospective case series. The description is given in table 1.

The anatomical districts with related pathologies treated as described with BMAC are illustrated in table 2. In particular, knee and hip joints treated with BMAC, including intraarticular

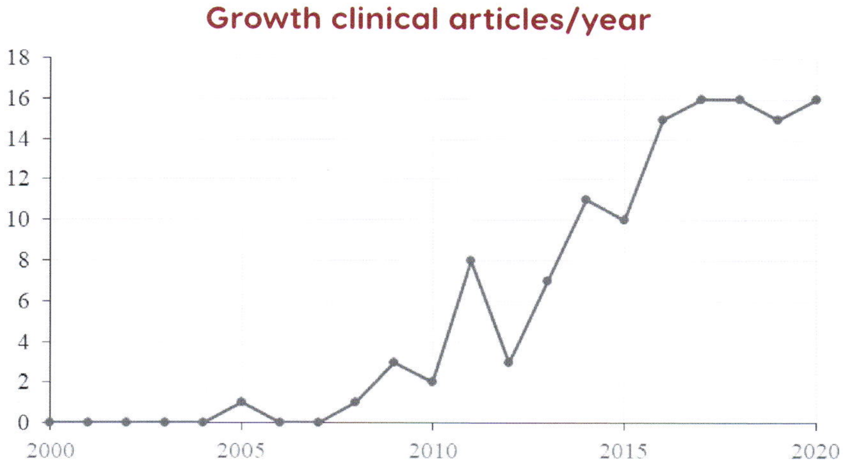

Figure 2 Cumulative annual growth 2000-2020 clinical articles with BMAC for musculoskeletal applications

Table 1 Distribution of studies by type (level of evidence).

Type of study	Number of studies
Randomized controlled trials (liv. I-II)	17
Prospective controlled studies (liv. III)	15
Series of prospective cases/control case (liv. IV)	45
Series of retrospective cases (liv. IV)	47
Total	**124**

therapy treatment of chondral and osteochondral defects, represented the most treated districts.

Overall, were included in the surveys 4,735 patients, 3,900 of whom received BMAC treatment under various conditions: BMAC only, BMAC in combination with PRP, BMAC in combination with heterologous, homologous, or synthetic *scaffolds*.

The mean age (±SD) of enrolled patients was 44.2±14.5 years (*range* 4-87), and mean *follow-up* (±SD) was 26.4±25.9 months (*range* 2-216). The

Table 2 Distribution of studies by anatomical district, including patients and patients who have received BMAC treatment.

Anatomical district	Number of studies	Total number of patients included in the studies	Total number of patients treated with BMAC
Knee	33 (26,6%)	1.727	1.378
Traumatology	19 (15,3%)	462	363
Ankle	18 (14,5%)	805	581
Avascular osteonecrosis (hip/knee)	15 (12,1%)	909	837
Cranio-maxillofacial	13 (10,4%)	101	91
Spine	10 (8,1%)	245	239
Shoulder/tendon	6 (4,8%)	269	212
Meniscus/LCA reconstruction	4 (3,2%)	35	35
Hip	2 (1,6%)	9	9
Tennis elbow	1 (0,8%)	30	30
Other	3 (2,4%)	125	125
Total	**124**	**4.735**	**3900**

bone marrow aspirate was mainly taken from the anterior and posterior iliac wings. Other sampling sites were: vertebral body, proximal tibia, iliac bone, proximal humerus, distal femur. The average volume of bone marrow aspirate taken corresponded to 81.6±73.4 mL (*range* 13-400) and the average volume of BMAC applied was 10.6±11.2 mL, with an average concentration of 9.0±4.1x. No significant adverse events were recorded in the assembly, confirming that the procedure was safe.

Analysis of the results showed proven efficacy (results evaluated overall positive by the authors) in 105 studies (84.7%),12 articles (9.7%) reported results without statistically significant differences to control groups or pre-intervention conditions. In contrast, 7 authors (5.6%) concluded by expressing a negative opinion with respect to BMAC treatment. Negative results were referred to three treatments with BMAC in avascular necrosis of the femoral head, one treatment in vertebral surgery, one treatment in craniomaxillofacial surgery, one treatment of cartilage defect of the knee, one treatment for post-traumatic osteoarthritis of the ankle, and one treatment following diaphyseal trauma.

Eighty-seven out of 124 articles described the system used for the concentration of bone marrow aspirate. Table 3 shows the details of the systems used (CE marked or FDA registered) with the relevant manufacturer. Regarding the evaluation of efficacy, the 5 most frequently used concentration systems were considered as described in the articles in the materials and methods section, which were respectively: the BMAC device - Harvest/Terumo (fig. 3a), BioCUE - Zimmer-Biomet (fig. 3b), Magellan - Isto-Biologics/Arteriocyte (fig. 3c), Angel - Arthrex (fig. 3d) and Res-Q60 BMC IOR-G1 - Novagenit/Thermogenesis (fig. 3e).

The evaluation parameters taken into account were related to the content within the BMAC of nucleated cells (TNC, *Total Nucleated Cells*), *mononuclear cells* (MNC), non-hematopoietic progenitor cells CFU-F (*Colony Forming Unit-Fibroblast*), of the CD34+ hematopoietic line cells and platelets (PLT), compared to the midollar aspi-

Table 3 Systems used for the concentration of bone marrow aspirate.

Device (trade name)	Manufacturer/Distributor	Number of studies where used
BMAC®	Harvest/Terumo	34 (39%)
BioCUE®	Zimmer-Biomet	11 (13%)
Magellan	IstoBiologics/Arteriocyte	10 (11%)
Angel®	Arthrex	6 (7%)
Res-Q™60 BMC IOR-G1	Novagenit	4 (5%)
Sepax®	Biosafe	4 (5%)
ART-BMC	Celling Bioscience	3 (3%)
PureBMC®	Emcyte	2 (2%)
Others	-	13 (15%)
Total		**87**

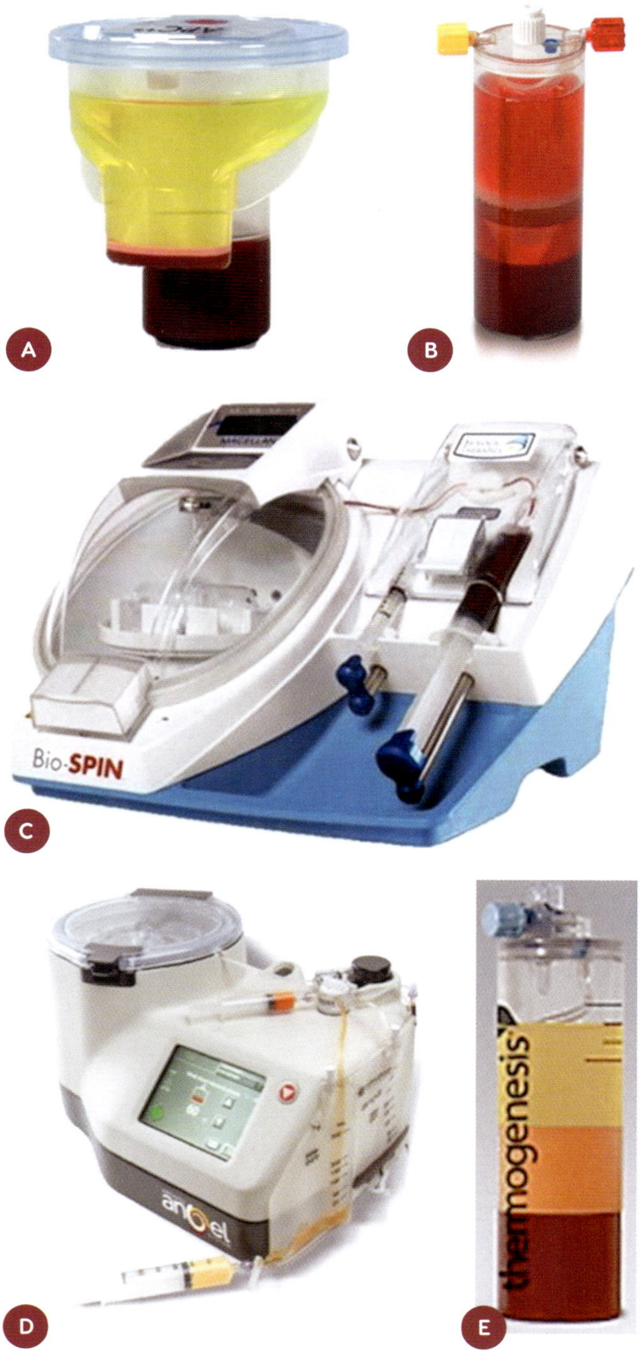

Figure 3 More frequent bone marrow aspirate concentration systems used and reported in the literature analysis: BMAC-Harvest/Therumo (a); BioCue-Zimmer/Biomet (b); Magellan-IstoBiologics/Arteriocyte (c); Angel-Arthrex (d); IOR-G1 ResQ 60 Novagenit/Thermogenesis (e)

rate before processing. These criteria were not reported for all systems in a detailed and homogeneous manner within the articles, and no comparative studies comparing all concentration devices were detected. The manufacturers' web pages where it was possible to *download White Papers* elaborated by researchers who claimed to have received sponsorships from the companies and who compared a limited number of systems were then consulted. The authors concluded that, although a comparison from a technological point of view may indicate differences between the systems (e.g., distribution of BMAC fractions automatically, minimum concentrated volume, filtration accessories), the same cannot be said for the chondrogenic or anti-arthritic power of BMAC due to insufficient cellular characterization [9].

In addition to the literature, the commercial dissemination documentation (monographs, *brochures*, etc.) was consulted and the data, in some cases, were divergent from the articles referring to the same device. It was therefore considered, concerning the values reported in the literature and the available documentation, to calculate for each device an average value for each evaluation index resulting from the quantitative and qualitative analysis of each BMAC obtained from the processing, with a volume of concentrate between 4 and 10 mL and with hematocrit values between 7 and 11%. The data are summarised in table 4.

Table 4 Parameters compared for each system in terms of increased concentration (x from baseline) and cell recovery (%).

Device (trade name)	TNC	MNC	CFU-F	CD34+	PLT
BMAC®	4,9x (62%)	4.9x (69%)	4.8x (82%)	5.0x (78%)	6.0x (66%)
BioCUE®	6.3x (78%)	6.9x (80%)	5.9 (49%)	6,5x (72%)	7,4x (82%)
Magellan	4.0x (39%)	5.0x (39%)	6.0x (35%)	5.4x (-)	6.0 (56%)
Angel®	6.3x (76%)	6.5x (72%)	4,9x (44%)	7.0x (38%)	8x (58%)
Res-Q™60 IOR-G1	6.2x (73%)	6.0x (79%)	6,1x (80%)	6.9x (96%)	7x (78%)

From the technical data analyzed available in the literature and from the evaluations based on the analysis of the dissemination material, it can be said that overall a substantial equivalence of the five major BMAC systems used in terms of performance (concentration x) prevails with respect to the baseline BMA, in particular with regard to some benchmarks such as TNC content (4.0x-5.3x range), MNC (4.9x-6.5x range), CFU-F (4.8x-6.1x range), CD34+ (5.0x-7.0x range) and PLT (6.0x-8.0x range)) while a significant variability was recorded in terms of cellular recovery whose values were respectively: TNC *range* 39%-78%, MNC 39%-80%, CFU-F range 35%-82%, CD34+ *range* 38%-96%, PLT *range* 56%-82%. However, from the technological point of view, it is understood that the principle of gravitational separation based on the different specific gravity of each of the components of the bone marrow blood unites all the devices, the various systems differ in the ability to isolate the buffy coat in a more or less selective way, in particular the content of nucleated cells (TNC) and platelets (PLT), limiting the content of erythrocytes and neutrophils as much as possible. Capture chambers, cytometric reading systems, devices that allow automatic separation, and sensors based on the turbidimetric principle represented some of the peculiarities of the concentration devices of the bone marrow aspirate. Some systems have the advantage of closed-circuit processing, thus limiting the risk of contamination.

So far, the concentration systems of the bone marrow aspirate have been analyzed, which, as highlighted, did not differ significantly from the procedures reported in the instructions (all recommend a centrifugation speed included in the range 2,200 - 3,500 rpm for a time between 10 and 15 minutes) and for the final volume of concentrate and its cellular (TNC) and platelet (PLT) contents.

From a clinical point of view, almost 85% of the articles reported positive results with proven therapeutic benefits. However, the percentage of randomized and controlled investigations was limited (13.7%) compared to the total of the studies examined, and in the conclusions, the authors reiterated the need for further clinical evidence. These systems have shown advantages, are easy to use, and, considering the minimal manipulation that the cell population faces, do not present regulatory obstacles considering that most are FDA-approved or bear CE marking. In addition to the undifferentiated mesenchymal cell population, BMAC includes growth factors in the PLT fraction, particularly PDGF, TGF-β and BMP-2, and BMP-7, which is known to possess anabolic and anti-inflammatory effects [10]. In addition, the literature reports that BMAC has a significant concentration of interleukin-1 antagonist receptors, particularly IL-1RA [11]. This molecule inhibits the catabolism of IL-1 and, therefore, can play a decisive role in the attenuation of painful symptoms [12].

Evolution

From the general evaluations, it can be concluded that the use of BMAC, now considered a *Point of Care*, represents from a clinical point of view a practical regenerative approach to the treatment of diseases of the musculoskeletal system. Can we, however, as mentioned, consider it a *Standard of Care*? The literature points out that some limits persist referring to the processing/preparation of BMAC, in particular to the presence of aggregates capable of incorporating a certain amount of MSCs and HSCs, which when eliminated by filtration and centrifugation, can reduce the content of progenitor cells within the concentrate [13].

In addition, some authors attribute to centrifugation a potential loss of progenitor cells after bone marrow sampling, following an increase in the volumetric nucleus/cytoplasm ratio of the nucleated cells and with a consequent sedimentation together with red blood cells [14]. Others argue that there is a need for greater cellular characterization to minimize as much as possible the content of red blood cells from peripheral blood during the bone marrow sampling maneuver. It has been shown that erythrocytes during sampling or centrifugation can go into apoptosis. The resulting hemolysis releases toxic forms of hemoglobin capable of generating oxidative stress and releasing pro-inflammatory factors such as the macrophage migration inhibition factor (MIF) considered potent cytokine [15]. In summary, all these risks inhibit the regeneration potential of mesenchymal cells, therefore, reducing the clinical efficacy of BMAC in the treatment of diseases affecting the musculoskeletal system. Finally, it has been shown that this detail can influence even more the clinical outcome in the case of intra-articular intraarticular therapy [16, 9]. Consequently, the research in the field of regenerative medicine in the orthopedic field has continued to show a certain evolutionary dynamics; *in vitro* studies report improvements in terms of yield and cellular characterization thanks to new bone marrow concentration systems or even, going further, propose procedures that do not provide for the concentration of the bone marrow aspirate by centrifugation, such as the use of particular devices (suction trocars) (fig. 4) able, through specific sampling maneuvers from the site, to obtain reduced volumes of bone marrow aspirate but with a content of progenitor cell population (CFU-F) qualitatively higher, minimizing the infiltration of periph-

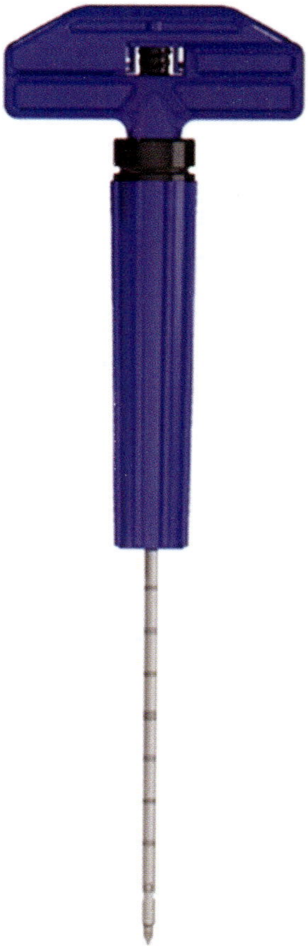

Figure 4 Trocar (Marrow Cellution) for autologous medullary aspirate sampling

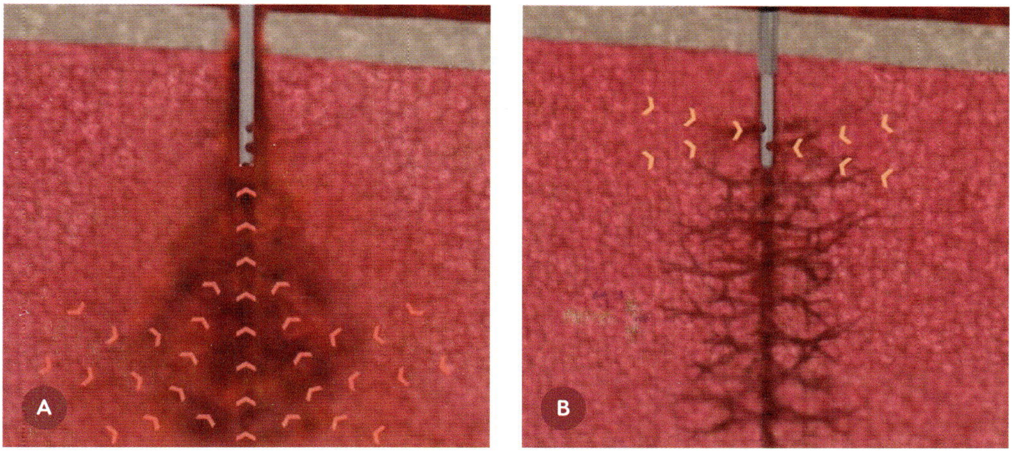

Figure 5 Traditional system of sampling of autologous bone marrow aspirate with aspiration through opening at the distal end of the device (a). Innovative trocar end with side openings that allow to reduce the infiltration of peripheral blood (b)

eral blood thanks to particular geometries (lateral openings)
compared to traditional sampling trocars with openings located at the end (fig. 5a and 5b). It has been shown that a system approved for clinical use allows sampling of 10 mL of BMA and has a substantial equivalence with respect to the use of BMAC. These systems claim ease of use, significantly reduced times from the moment of withdrawal to the administration to the patient of the aspirate, and regenerative potential higher than BMAC [17]. In small numbers and with short follow-ups, clinical investigations where the therapeutic efficacy is demonstrated using these devices in particular in joint infiltrative therapy for osteoarthritis of the knee [18] and in the primary arthroscopic revision of previous treatment of rotator cuff injuries [19] are described.
Similarly to systems that do not require centrifugation, other innovations are being developed clinically: the Stem-G2 (Novagenit) system, for example, takes up the principle of bone marrow blood sampling through precise maneuvers. Moreover, being

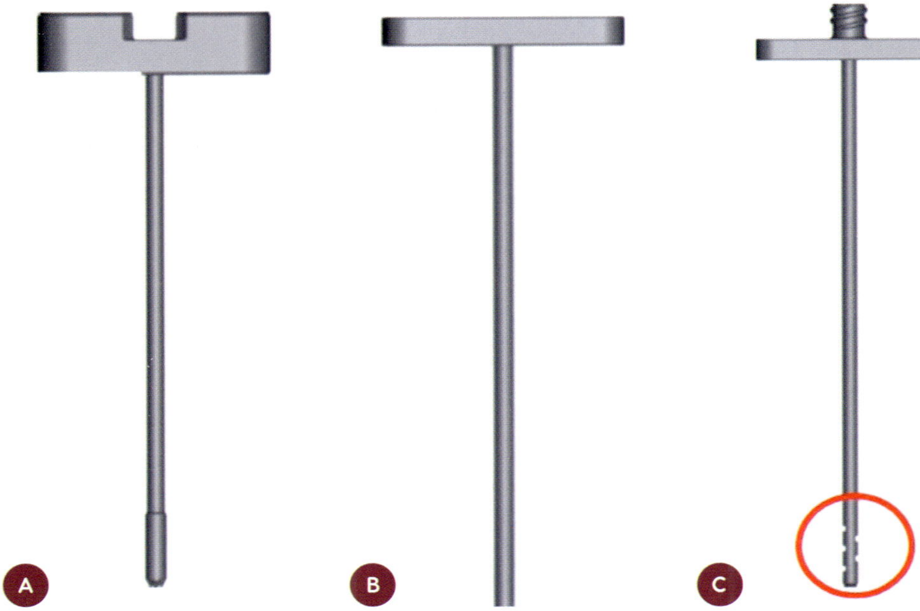

Figure 6 STEM-G2 bone marrow aspirated sampling system. Trocar guide (a); Spindle (b); Blind bottom suction cannula with side holes positioned at 180° for suction (c).

the blind-bottomed cannula equipped with lateral windows, it prevents infiltration of peripheral blood (fig. 6). Clinical trials are currently underway to validate this technology.

Conclusions

Concentrated bone marrow aspirate, as it has been known for some time, has a high regenerative potential and can be effectively used in the treatment of diseases affecting the musculoskeletal system thanks to the regenerative effect and paracrine action of specific progenitor cell populations. However, this literature analysis has helped to better understand some important aspects that should not be overlooked, such as the identification of the sampling site, the uniformity of the treatment protocols, the type of subject to be treated, and the age.

The bibliography confirms that the iliac wing (anterior and posterior) remains the anatomical sampling district of choice given the high clinically relevant concentration of progenitor cells compared to other sites such as the proximal tibia, the vertebral body, the distal femur, and the proximal humerus. All systems are equipped with sampling trocars that minimize the invasiveness of the procedure. The selection of patients is an equally important aspect; it is necessary to avoid creating false expectations, particularly in subjects of advanced age, while nevertheless recognizing the therapy's potentially anti-inflammatory purposes in this population segment. Another critical factor is the suitability of the therapy. It should be reiterated that this regenerative approach does not represent an alternative to repair, but in some diseases, it procrastinates over time more invasive interventions (i.e., cartilage damage). In others, it proves to be an effective solution in the regeneration of permanently compromised tissues (e.g., pseudoarthrosis). Of course, the general clinical conditions of the subject to be treated and the collaboration of the same in compliance with the rehabilitation protocol should not be neglected.

Finally, the prospect of new technologies that could accelerate procedures with a lower volume of bone marrow sampling, leaving out the steps of filtration and centrifugation and isolating the progenitor cell population in a more particular way, is certainly fascinating and can open up new therapeutic opportunities. Beyond the media/commercial aspect, the results of preliminary clinical investigations are promising. However, some aspects and questions are still to be explored and can only be answered through scientific evidence resulting from rigorous prospective and controlled clinical investigations.

References

1. Brittberg M, Lindahl A, Nilsson A, Ohlsson C, Isaksson O, Peterson L. Treatment of deep cartilage defects in the knee with autologous chondrocyte transplantation. N Engl J Med. 1994;331:889-95.
2. Bartlett W, Gooding CR, Carrington RW, Skinner JA, Briggs TW, Bentley G. Autologous chondrocyte implantation at the knee using a bilayer collagen membrane with bone graft. A preliminary report, J

Bone Joint Surg Br. 2005;87(3):330-332.
3. Vannini F, Cavallo M, Ramponi L, Castagnini F, Massimi S, Giannini S, Buda RE. Return to Sports After Bone Marrow-Derived Cell Transplantation for Osteochondral Lesions of the Talus. Cartilage. 2017;8(1):80-87.
4. Turner L, Knoepfler P. Selling Stem Cells in the USA: Assessing the Direct-to-Consumer Industry. Cell Stem Cell. 2016;19(2):154-157.
5. Frost& Sullivan. Geographical Overview for Regenerative Medicine Company. Sep. 2015
6. Alvarez-Viejo M, Menendez-Menendez Y, Blanco-Gelaz MA, Ferrero-Gutierrez A, Fernandez-Rodriguez MA, Gala J, Otero-Hernandez J. Quantifying mesenchymal stem cells in the mononuclear cell fraction of bone marrow samples obtained for cell therapy. Transplant Proc. 2013;45(1):434-9.
7. Kaplan A. Review: mesenchymal stem cells: cell-based reconstructive therapy in orthopaedics. Tissue Eng. 2005;11(7-8):1198-211.
8. Everts PA, Malanga GA, Paul RW, Rothenberg GB, Stephens N, Mautner KR. Assessing clinical implications and perspectives of the pathophysiological effects of erythrocytes and plasma free haemoglobin in autologous biologics for use in musculoskeletal regenerative medicine therapies. A review. Regenerative Therapy. 2019;11:56-64.
9. Gaul F, Bugbee WD, Hoenecke HR, D'Lima DD. A Review of Commercially Available Point-of-Care Devices to Concentrate Bone Marrow for the Treatment of Osteoarthritis and Focal Cartilage Lesions. Cartilage. 2019;10(4):387-394.
10. Schnabel LV, Mohammed HO, Miller BJ, McDermott WG, Jacobson MS, Santangelo KS, Fortier LA. Platelet Rich Plasma (PRP) Enhances Anabolic Gene Expression Patterns in Flexor Digitorum Superficialis Tendons. J Orthop Res. 2007;25(2):230-40.
11. Cassano JM, Kennedy JG, Ross KA, Fraser EJ, Goodale MB, Fortier LA. Bone marrow concentrate and platelet-rich plasma differ in cell distribution and interleukin 1 receptor antagonist protein concentration. Knee Surg Sports Traumatol Arthrosc. 2018; 26(1):333-342.
12. Wehling P, Moser C, Frisbie D, et al. Autologous conditioned serum in the treatment of orthopedic diseases: The orthokine therapy. Biodrugs. 2007;21:323-332.
13. Bhartiya D, Shaikh A, Nagvenkar P, et al. Very small embryonic-like stem cells with maximum regenerative potential get discarded during cord blood banking and bone marrow processing for autologous stem cell therapy. Stem cells and development. 2012;21:1-6.
14. Zuba-Surma EK, Kucia M, Ratajczak J, Ratajczak MZ. "Small stem cells" in adult tissues: very small embryonic-like stem cells stand up! Cytometry. 2009;75:4-13.
15. Xiong C, Huang B, Zhou Y, Cun YP, Liu LT, Wang J, et al. Macrophage migration inhibitory factor inhibits the migra-

tion of cartilage end plate-derived stem cells by reacting with CD74. PLoS One. 2012;7(8):e43984.
16. Braun HJ, Kim HJ, Chu CR, Dragoo JL. The effect of platelet rich plasma formulations and blood products on human synoviocytes: Implications for intraarticular injury and therapy. Am J Sports Med. 2014;42(5):1204-10.
17. Scarpone M, Kuebler D, Chambers A, De Filippo CM, Amatuzio M, Ichim TE, Patel AN, Caradonna E. Isolation of clinically relevant concentrations of bone marrow mesenchymal stem cells without centrifugation. J Transl Med. 2019 Jan 5;17(1):10.
18. Varady NH, Cate G, Barghi A, Jobe N, Yakin B, Ylanan RC, Arnold CA. Positive early clinical outcomes of bone marrow aspirate concentrate for osteoarthritis using a novel fenestrated trocar. Knee. 2020;27(5):1627-1634.
19. The Influence of Trocar Fenestration and Volume on Connective Tissue Progenitor Cells (Stem Cells) in Arthroscopic Bone Marrow Aspiration From the Proximal Humerus. Arthroscopy. 2017;33(6):1167-1174.

CHAPTER 12

HY TISSUE PRP PLUS: MEDICAL DEVICE FOR AUTOLOGOUS PRP

Carlo Soranzo[1], Alessia Tognetto[1], Luis Vidal[2]

1) Fidia Farmaceutici SpA, Abano Terme, Italy

2) Laboratorios Fidia Farmaceutica, Madrid, Spain

Introduction

Tissue regeneration is still a therapeutic challenge, even if different therapeutic approaches are now being studied. It is likely that a potential approach to tissue healing in a regenerative sense consists in the administration of multi-molecular preparations capable of satisfying the entire complexity of biological *signaling*, providing the environmental stimuli necessary to regulate the intrinsic regenerative mechanisms. In this sense, Platelet Rich Plasma (PRP) has emerged as a possible therapeutic option in regenerative medicine. The rationale and characterization studies of the first PRP preparations began in the hematological field in the mid-70s to describe a transfusion product intended for the treatment of patients with thrombocytopenia. About ten years later, PRP began to be used in maxillofacial surgery as Platelet-Rich Fibrin (PRF), and in 2001, Marx defined PRP as a volume of autologous plasma with a platelet concentration above baseline [1]. Since then, PRP has been used for tissue regeneration within various pathologies in different specialties, including dentistry, orthopedics and sports medicine, plastic surgery, and ophthalmology.

Although PRP is mainly composed of platelets and plasma (optionally, leukocytes can be included in the preparations, but their therapeutic role is still debated today), platelets are the characterizing element to a large extent, since they contribute, thanks to their complex molecular composition, to the important biological activity ascribed to the PRP. Megakaryocytes produce these anucleated discoid cellular elements in the bone marrow under the hormonal control of thrombopoietin. The physiological count of circulating platelets in the bloodstream ranges from 150,000 to 400,000 platelets per μ L with a half-life in the bloodstream of 7-10 days. Platelets contain three types of secretory granules: lysosomes, dense granules, and alpha granules, the latter being the most abundant group.

The primary function of platelets in the regulation of hemostasis and coagulation. Following a vascular lesion, platelets are activated and promote the formation of the clot. Platelet activation induces the release of several growth factors (GFS) from α granules such as PDGF, TFG-β, EGF, VEGF, IGF, and various others, which exert their physiological functions as a stimulus to the healing of injured tissue.

Therefore, the concept behind the therapeutic use of PRP is simple. Since platelets are a significant source of trophic factors within blood clots, the idea of concentrating platelets at the site of injury could speed up and optimize the healing process. Therefore, by conveying more platelets to a potentially injured tissue, the concentration of deposed trophic factors and other biological stimuli of platelet derivation, which activate the healing process in a regenerative sense, also increases. Therefore, the use of PRP has gradually extended to the treatment of various pathological conditions, both chronic and acute.

Effects of PRP

Autologous PRP treatment soon highlighted the ability to modulate inflammation and stimulate repair at the application site. As already mentioned, the mechanism underlying the therapeutic activity of PRP is the release of a vast *array* of signaling molecules, including growth factors (GF) and chemokines, locally at the site of injury. In short, the biological components released by PRP are able to interfere with the microenvironment of the lesion, modulating the inflammatory response, inducing cell migration and proliferation, and regulating angiogenesis and cell differentiation. The PRP's ordered activation of these biological processes can determine the so-called tissue healing in a regenerative sense and confer a clinical benefit. Below there are some experimental evidences to support this claim:

- Activation of cell migration, proliferation, and differentiation processes: in vitro, PRP stimulates chemotaxis and cell proliferation. PRP induces cell motility by inducing changes in the cytoskeleton of human osteoblasts, increases migration, and stimulates the differentiation in a chondrogenic sense of human subchondral progenitor cells grown in high-density pellets, or of mesenchymal stem cells (MSCs) or mesenchymal stem cells of adipocyte derivation (ADSCs);

- Extracellular matrix synthesis (ECM): In vitro studies have shown that PRP stimulates chondrocytes to produce the cartilaginous matrix while controlling the synthesis of mediators of the inflammatory response, such as IL-1 β. In addition, PRP also increases the synthesis of proteoglycans and type II collagen, fundamental elements for the structural organization of the cartilaginous matrix. PRP's anabolic effect is closely linked to the promotion of TGF-β synthesis, a cytokine that reduces type I collagen synthesis and increases gene expression of type II collagen and aggrecan.
- Anti-inflammatory action: in vitro, PRP has demonstrated the ability to reverse the inflammatory response induced by IL-1 β of chondrocytes isolated from patients with osteoarthritis, including the activation of NFϰB. Similarly, always in chondrocytes or synoviocytes of arthritic patients, PRP is able to neutralize the transcription induced by IL-1 β of the genes encoding ADAMTS4 and COX2.
- Angiogenesis: PRP can induce proliferation, migration, and formation of tubular structures in human umbilical endothelial cells. Recently, Levoux et al. [2] have shown that, after activation, platelets can transfer mitochondria, functionally competent for the respiratory chain, to MSCs in close contact with them by exocytosis. Subsequently, such platelet-derived mitochondria promote the pro-angiogenic activity of MSCs through their metabolic remodeling. The possibility of transferring cellular organelles, and not only trophic factors and/or soluble mediators, to target cells may open a new, important chapter in platelet biology and the therapeutic function of PRP.
- Analgesia: PRP exerts a powerful anti-nociceptive activity linked, at least in part, to the induction of endocannabinoids and related compounds (analgesic mediators), in particular in the tissues hosting active inflammatory processes.

Role of erythrocytes (RBCs) in PRP

Since it has been noted that the presence of red blood cells in the joint is associated with cartilage damage, some authors believe that exposure of articular cartilage to whole blood is to be avoided. It has been shown that it causes the inhibition of proteoglycan synthesis, the death of chondrocytes, the stimulation of metalloprotease secretion (MMP), and the formation of hydroxyl radicals (probably a function of the amount of hemoglobin, and therefore ferrous ion, present) in the vicinity of chondrocytes, producing an irreversible harmful effect at the level of cartilage matrix. For this reason, PRP must be poor in red blood cells.

PRP classification and preparation systems

There are several methods to obtain PRP, but basically, all of them consist of centrifuging a certain amount (however, less than 60ml if the procedure is carried out outside a transfusion center) of peripheral venous blood, separating the platelet-rich plasma fraction. Based on the terminologies of some authors, the efficiency and characteristics of the processes and attributes of the finished PRP product, different classification systems for PRP formulations have been published. However, a general consensus on the PRP classification system has never been reached. Ideally, a classification system should focus on the characteristics of the product and the most appropriate nomenclature to describe the therapeutic process related to the patient's clinical condition. To date, however, the most used classification is based on the number of leukocytes contained in the finished product and the method of preparation. In other words, we speak of leukocyte-rich PRP (Leukocyte Rich-PRP) or leukocyte-poor PRP (Leukocyte Poor-PRP) depending on whether the concentration of leukocytes is higher or lower than the blood concentration. Another way to classify the different production methods of PRP is based on the number of centrifugations employed in the process, i.e., single or double centrifugation methods. Blood components can be fractionated using gravitational centrifugation techniques and devices. Centrifugation-based systems separate whole blood according to the specific densities of the various components, generally obtaining three fractions: red blood cells, plasma, and *buffy coats*. The *buffy coat* contains platelets and white blood cells/leukocytes (GB). In the single centrifugation protocol, the plasma fraction containing mainly platelets in high concentration is recovered as PRP. In the double centrifugation protocol, on the other hand, the entire fraction of plasma containing platelets is recovered and centrifuged again in a new tube to obtain a more concentrated PRP product.

Hy-Tissue PRP Plus

Each PRP kit produces platelet-rich plasma with specific concentration, yield, and purity characteristics. Hy-Tissue PRP Plus (Fidia Farmaceutici, Abano Terme, Padova) is a new, promising kit for obtaining PRP (intended for autologous use) with double centrifugation (fig 1). The system is a disposable medical device for outpatient and surgical use, which allows the process of 2 0ml of anticoagulated blood and obtaining autologous PRP with a high concentration of platelets in a closed system, mainly intended

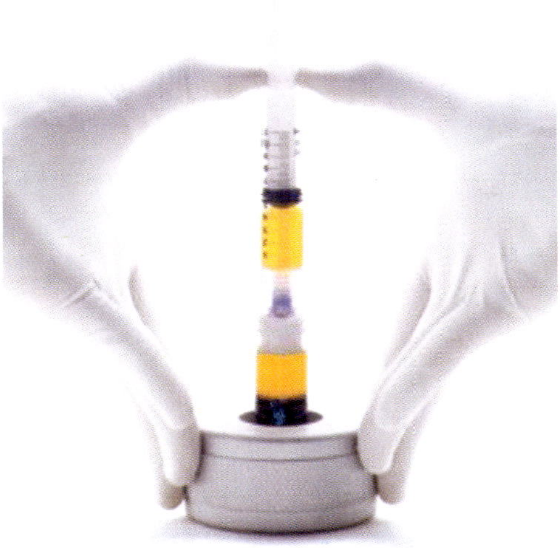

Figure 1 Laminar flow selection system allows the precise separation of the plasma fraction of PRP directly from the syringe in asepsis and in the absence of platelet activation

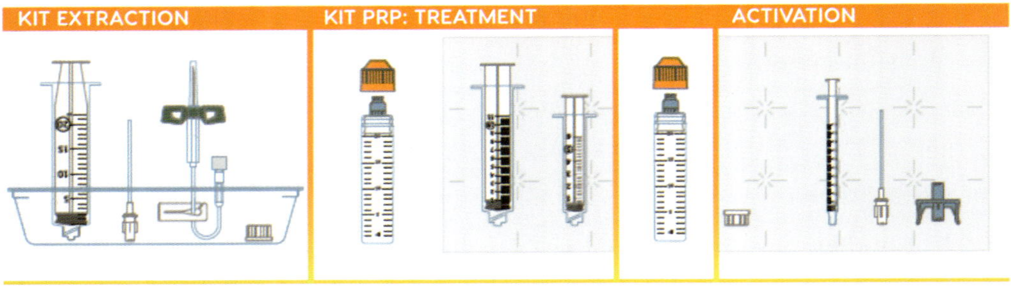

Figure 2 Composition of Hy Tissue PRP Plus kit. Extraction: tray with material for venous blood sampling, including filter cannula for the addition of anticoagulant solution (supplied separately). PRP Treatment Kit: syringes and tubes to carry out the two processing cycles. Activation Kit (optional): syringe and connectors to activate the platelet concentrate with 10% Solution of $CaCl_2$

for musculoskeletal and skin applications. The kit contains all the elements to carry out the complete processing, namely the material to operate the blood sampling, the sterile cylindrical containers with low cellular adhesiveness and patented to conduct the centrifugation and separation of plasma fractions in conditions of asepsis, as well as the reagents necessary for the preparation and activation of PRP (fig 2). The PRP obtained is activated with a solution of calcium chloride (1:20) to initiate degranulation, i.e., the release of the GFs contained in the platelet granules before infiltration to the site of injury.

Quality characteristics of PRP obtained with Hy-Tissue PRP Plus

A characterization study was performed at the Laboratory for the Preparation of Blood Components and Regenerative Medicine - Transfusion Medicine (Azienda Ospedaliera SS Antonio e Biagio, Alessandria) involving 20 donors, taking for each 20 ml of anticoagulated venous blood (18ml blood + 2ml solution of ACD-A). The taken blood (20 ml) was transferred in asepsis in the first separation device (fig 3A, 3B), following the instructions for use. It was centrifuged (1800 rpm,

8 min, 450G) using a dedicated centrifuge (Duografter II, Fidia Farmaceutici), obtaining the separation of the hematocrit (lower fraction) and the entire plasma fraction (upper) in which the platelets had concentrated (PRP1, fig 3C). Note that the *buffy coat* is not selected. This is possible thanks to the incredible precision with which the two layers can be separated by the mobile collection system (fig 3D).

The plasma was transferred to a second tube (fig 3E) and subjected to further centrifugation (2000 rpm, 10 min, 600G) which induced the sedimentation of the platelets at the bottom of the container. Finally, part of the platelet-poor plasma was removed (i.e., the PPP), and the platelet pellet was gently resuspended to obtain the fraction called PRP2 (Fig 3F) with a platelet concentration 4-6 times higher than the baseline value in the blood. Table 1 shows the evaluated hematological parameters: platelet concentration factor (PLT CF), platelet yield (PLT yield), as well as assessment of white blood cell (WBC) and erythrocyte (RBC) load.

As shown in the table, the absolute platelet count of the PRP2 fraction

Table 1 Mean values and standard deviation (SD) of the critical parameters used to characterize the PRP obtained through the Hy Tissue PRP Plus kit.

	Whole blood (baseline)	PRP2 Fraction
Vol (mL)	20.0 ± 0.0	3.0 ± 0.3
WBC (x10^6 cells/mL)	5.0 ± 0.9	3.3 ± 1.7
RBC (x10^9 cells/mL)	4.0 ± 0.3	0.01 ± 0.00
PLT (x10^6cells/mL)	190.7 ± 17.9	891.2 ± 88.6
PLT (resa %)	-	71 ± 9.9
PLT CF (x)	-	4.7 ± 0.6
Composition (%)		
PLT	-	98.5
WBC	-	0.4
RBC	-	1.1

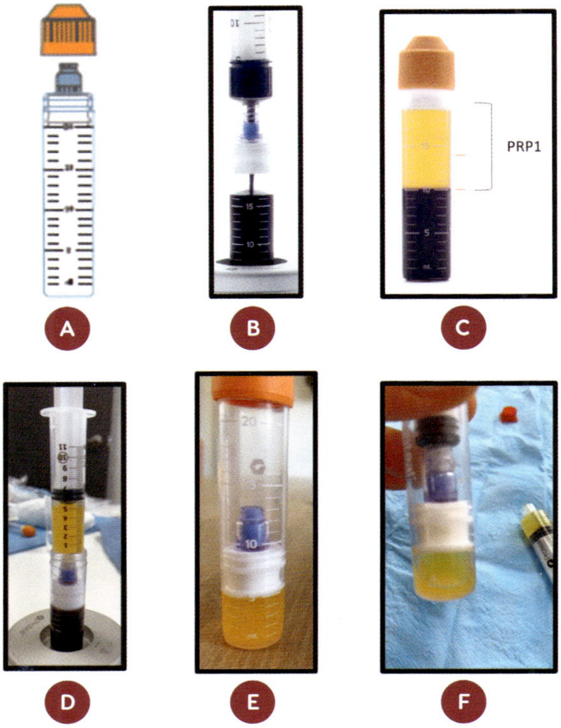

Figure 3 (A) Schematic drawing of the differential centrifugation tube. The neutral pressure valve with a lure-lock connection ensures the hermetic connection syringe – tube. The connection is open (inlet/outlet fluid) only when the union between the needle and the valve is correct. This ensures the transfer of blood or its derivatives into asepsis without risk of platelet activation.
(B) After blood sampling (anticoagulant), the same is transferred within the tube by connection to the valve as mentioned above, the processing volume is 20ml (18ml blood + 2ml anticoagulant solution).
(C) The blood is centrifuged under standard validated conditions (1800 rpm, 450G: P cycle). The different blood components are separated by centrifugal force. In this cycle, the entire plasma fraction is isolated, i.e., the sovereign fraction of straw color, clouded by the presence of platelets (PRP1). Selecting the 2ml below the demarcation boundary of the plasma with the red lower phase collects the fraction called "buffy coat."
(D) The PRP1 fraction is recovered by means of a push-out system, which allows the transfer in asepsis of fluids between the two compartments (tube – syringe)
(E) The PRP1 fraction is transferred to a second tube and centrifuged (2000rpm, 600G: L cycle) in order to concentrate the platelets at the bottom of the container; while the superior plasma fraction (about 2/3 of the total volume) is discarded (PPP fraction)
(F) Platelets weakly aggregated to the bottom are gently resuspended with a rotary movement. This results in an average of 3 mL of PRP (or PRP2 fraction) with a platelet concentration in the range of 1,000,000 PLT/mL ± 20 %

shows a concentration 5 times higher than the starting value, i.e., in compliance with legal requirements. It is reasonable to think that a greater platelet content corresponds to a greater amount of GFs and active substances brought locally and, therefore, a better clinical result. The presence, or not, of the leukocyte-rich fraction (buffy coat) should also be considered. PRP-containing white blood cells will have a different biological activity from PRP in which they are absent or in low quantities. It is generally accepted that the leukocyte cells present in the buffy coat exhibit a pro-inflammatory activity, compared to a PRP with a low leukocyte index (lower than the baseline value of the blood before treatment). HT PRP Plus allows you to precisely select the buffy coat, including it (LR-PRP with pro-inflammatory activity) or excluding it (LP-PRP without inflammatory activity, called for this "anti-inflammatory"). The buffy coat is that "red" fraction of about 1.5-2 ml below the level of the plasma fraction. HY Tissue PRP systems are CE-marked medical devices and have recently been approved by the US FDA using the 510k procedure and have recently begun commercialization in that market.

Clinical applications

There are many clinical applications of PRP in the orthopedic field, although further studies will be needed to demonstrate the full potential of this product. A further reason for the variability in the results is the poor characterization of the PRP used. The platelet content of the final preparation is not always indicated, as well as the presence or absence of the buffy coat and/or any erythrocyte contaminant. Saying that, however, PRP can be considered a valid alternative to different clinical situations in which more traditional approaches are no longer effective or if you want to associate PRP itself with more established therapies to maximize its effect.

Epicondylitis

PRP was studied as a treatment option

for patients with lateral epicondylitis who did not respond to physical therapy. Mishra (Mishra et al. 2014) evaluated 230 patients in a prospective cohort study who did not respond to at least 3 months of conservative treatment for lateral epicondylitis. PRP injection was associated with a significant improvement in pain at 24 weeks (71.5% vs. 56.1%, p = 0.019). Other studies have suggested that PRP may relieve pain and associated symptoms longer than injecting corticosteroids[3].

Patellar tendinopathy

PRP was useful in chronic refractory patellar tendinopathy compared to shock wave therapy [4].

Achilles' tendinopathy

Achilles tendinopathy is one of the most frequent injuries related to excessive use of the ankle joint. PRP injections produced good overall results for the treatment of chronic recalcitrant Achilles tendinopathy with a stable outcome up to a medium-term follow-up [5].

Rotator cuff lesions

A recent systematic review of randomized controlled clinical trials using the arthroscopic technique has shown that treatment with PRP translates, compared to control groups, into better cure rates and functional outcomes with less pain, especially in major lesions (>3 cm) [6].

Plantar fasciitis

With or without ultrasound guidance, PRP injections into the plantar fascia have been introduced as an alternative therapy to standard treatments. A recent meta-analysis reported that PRP is as effective as other treatments in reducing pain and improving function in patients with the condition, even superior to steroid treatments to relieve long-term pain [7].

Osteoarthrosis and knee cartilage defects

Clinical evidence for the use of PRP in the treatment of cartilage lesions in patients with osteoarthritis of the knee or hip is well established. Intra-articular injections of LP-PRP are now considered a safe treatment and able to reduce pain and improve function in patients diagnosed with osteoarthritis of the knee. In a group of such patients (KL grade II / III), Guillibert et al. [8] showed that a single injection of LP-PRP, produced using Hy-Tissue PRP, resulted in significant functional improvement and pain relief in 80% of patients, with benefits up to 6 months after injection. Similarly, Finogejevs et al. [9] confirmed that infiltration of LP-PRP (obtained thanks to the Hy-Tissue PRP kit) counteracts pain and improves knee function in patients with osteoarthritis up to 12 months after administration, better than with triamcinolone treatment.

Meniscal lesions

Meniscal injuries are still an unsolved problem in sports traumatology, and in the majority of cases, partial meniscectomy is the only treatment option. Unfortunately, the meniscus's removal, even partial, predisposes the knee joint to degenerative processes. A retrospective study with 10 patients with degenerative meniscal lesions without knee osteoarthritis was evaluated 6 months after intra-meniscal administration of Hy-Tissue PRP, resulting in an improvement in the KOOS score from 56.6 ± 15.7 to 72.7 ± 18.5 ($P = 0.0007$) [10].

Conclusion

In conclusion, the use of PRP requires that in the near future, further studies will be conducted to investigate its multiple therapeutic applications in the field of tissue regeneration and consolidate what has been demonstrated so far; however, already with the current evidence, this product has proven to be a valid therapeutic option in several fields, in particular in orthopedics.

References

1. Marx, R. E., Platelet-rich plasma (PRP): what is PRP and what is not PRP? *Implant Dent* 2001, *10* (4), 225-8.
2. Levoux, J.; Prola, A.; Lafuste, P.; Gervais, M.; Chevallier, N.; Koumaiha, Z.; Kefi, K.; Braud, L.; Schmitt, A.; Yacia, A.; Schir-

mann, A.; Hersant, B.; Sid-Ahmed, M.; Ben Larbi, S.; Komrskova, K.; Rohlena, J.; Relaix, F.; Neuzil, J.; Rodriguez, A. M., Platelets Facilitate the Wound-Healing Capability of Mesenchymal Stem Cells by Mitochondrial Transfer and Metabolic Reprogramming. *Cell Metab* 2020.

3. Gosens, T.; Peerbooms, J. C.; van Laar, W.; den Oudsten, B. L., Ongoing positive effect of platelet-rich plasma versus corticosteroid injection in lateral epicondylitis: a double-blind randomized controlled trial with 2-year follow-up. *Am J Sports Med* 2011, *39* (6), 1200-8.
4. Dragoo, J. L.; Wasterlain, A. S.; Braun, H. J.; Nead, K. T., Platelet-rich plasma as a treatment for patellar tendinopathy: a double-blind, randomized controlled trial. *Am J Sports Med* 2014, *42* (3), 610-8.
5. Filardo, G.; Kon, E.; Di Matteo, B.; Di Martino, A.; Tesei, G.; Pelotti, P.; Cenacchi, A.; Marcacci, M., Platelet-rich plasma injections for the treatment of refractory Achilles tendinopathy: results at 4 years. *Blood transfusion = Trasfusione del sangue* 2014, *12* (4), 533-540.
6. Hurley, E. T.; Lim Fat, D.; Moran, C. J.; Mullett, H., The Efficacy of Platelet-Rich Plasma and Platelet-Rich Fibrin in Arthroscopic Rotator Cuff Repair: A Meta-analysis of Randomized Controlled Trials. *Am J Sports Med* 2019, *47* (3), 753-761.
7. Ling, Y.; Wang, S., Effects of platelet-rich plasma in the treatment of plantar fasciitis: A meta-analysis of randomized controlled trials. *Medicine* 2018, *97* (37), e12110-e12110.
8. Guillibert, C.; Charpin, C.; Raffray, M.; Benmenni, A.; Dehaut, F. X.; El Ghobeira, G.; Giorgi, R.; Magalon, J.; Arniaud, D., Single Injection of High Volume of Autologous Pure PRP Provides a Significant Improvement in Knee Osteoarthritis: A Prospective Routine Care Study. *Int J Mol Sci* 2019, *20* (6).
9. Elksniņš-Finogejevs, A.; Vidal, L.; Peredistijs, A., Intra-articular platelet-rich plasma vs corticosteroids in the treatment of moderate knee osteoarthritis: a single-center prospective randomized controlled study with a 1-year follow up. *Journal of orthopaedic surgery and research* 2020, *15* (1), 257-257.
10. Guenoun, D.; Magalon, J.; de Torquemada, I.; Vandeville, C.; Sabatier, F.; Champsaur, P.; Jacquet, C.; Ollivier, M., Treatment of degenerative meniscal tear with intrameniscal injection of platelets rich plasma. *Diagn Interv Imaging* 2019.

CHAPTER 13

THE LIPOGEMS SYSTEM AND OTHER DEVICES FOR THE PROCESSING OF ADIPOSE TISSUE IN THE REGENERATIVE THERAPY OF THE MUSCULOSKELETAL SYSTEM

Carlo Tremolada
Image Regenerative Clinic, Milan

Adipose tissue as regenerative tissue

The adipose tissue (subcutaneous and visceral) is the largest organ of our body and has multiple structural and endocrine support functions. It also has a very rich network of capillary microvessels that actively par-ticipate in the self-repair processes of our body mainly because, as all the capillaries of every human tis-sue, they are rich of perycites (fig. 1), which represent the precursors of MSCs (mesenchymal stem cells), cellular elements particularly important in reparative mechanisms.

Even in past centuries, starting with military doctors in the Napoleonic army, fat had been used with con-troversial results as a dressing. However, it is only since the 80s, with the invention of the liposuction technique and its increasing success, that access to large quantities of tissue with more minor and less in-vasive techniques has made the lipofilling technique popular, which is nothing more than an autologous

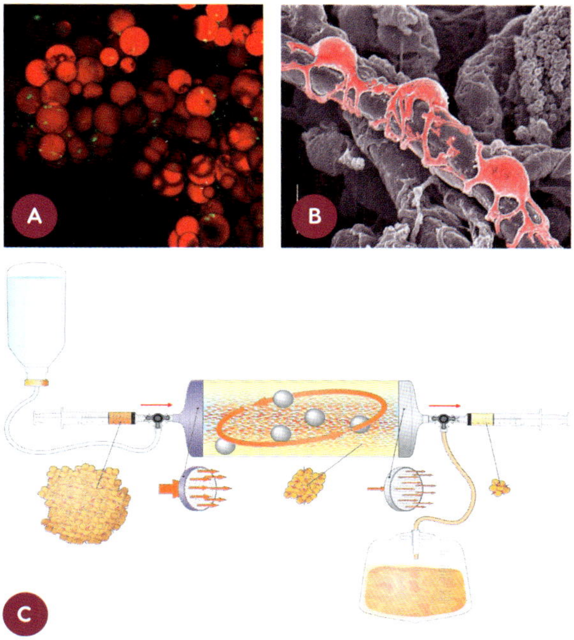

Figure 1 (A) Histological appearance of clusters of adipose tissue processed with lipogems technology (note the integrity of the adipocytes (orange spheres) and the presence of pericytes (small green cells in single file because they are present around the capillaries) (B) Appearance in electron microscopy of pericytes around a capillary. All vascularized tissues contain pericytes that detach in case of trauma and turn into MSCs that act as personalized micropharmacies secreting substances that initially regulate inflammation and later regeneration. (c) Lipogems technology. Essential is the processing in the absence of air that allows the protection of fat clusters that can be reduced while maintaining their integrity

transplant of adipose tissue with purposes initially aimed at restoring lost volumes (e.g., in breast recon-struction or facial defects) and later for regenerative purposes (in particular scars and radiodermatitis).

The biggest problems related to classical lipofilling techniques (also the most recent), alongside un-doubted clinical successes, are linked to the excessive variability of the results (volumetric resorption, ir-regularities, residual fibrosis, unpredictability in the regenerative result).

Comparison between adipose tissue and bone marrow aspirate as regenerative tissues and source of bio-logically and clinically active MSCs

Adipose tissue and bone marrow have become the most used tissues for "regenerative" purposes in the musculoskeletal system due to the ease and mini-traumatic of the withdrawal and the presence of MSCs in both aspirates. Bone marrow MSCs were, thanks to Arnold Caplan's studies and the fact that the bone marrow was well known as the progenitor organ of hematopoietic stem cells, the first to be studied, isolated, and charac-terized. However, the adipose tissue has shown to possess similar regenerative characteristics with some obvious advantages such as abundance, the even greater technical ease of the withdrawal, and a much more significant amount of obtainable mesenchymal stem cells [1].

The biological and clinical action of mesenchymal stem cells, as known, is mediated by their secretome that includes exosomes and proteins as well as RNA, so much so that Caplan himself has renamed them as "Medicinal Signaling Cell" with a biological action significant in the ordinary maintenance of tissues and the response to trauma. Mesenchymal stem cells derive from the pericytes of the capillaries of any tissue: trauma to the capillary wall causes the release in the tissue interstitium of the pericyte (PRP also works by stimulating the detachment of pericytes but has no effect on vascular density), which is a short time (minutes/ hours) turns into MSC and secretes numerous cytokines that interfere with inflammation and in particular with macrophages increasing its anti-inflammatory action; only after a couple of weeks numer-ous more specific cytokines are secreted with antibiotic, antifibrotic, angiogenetic and not least pain-relieving action. This field of medicine is booming with over 8,500 entries in the last year alone [2].

It is not clear what is the density of MSC necessary to obtain a specific biological action; however, the ex-cellent clinical action on symptomatic osteoarthritis of BMAC (concentrated bone marrow aspirate - about 20,000 MSC / cc) is comparable to one year to that of lipograms not concentrated but only praised whose average content is much higher (about 1,000,000 MSC / cc).

Withal, in the bone marrow aspiration, it is easier to count mesenchymal stem cells directly; in adipose tissue, direct counting is almost impossible as most mesenchymal stem cells are trapped in the mi-crovessels present within the tissue micro-clusters.

The count of mesenchymal stem cells in adipose tissue is possible only after an enzymatic or mechanical separation procedure that causes the complete (enzymatic) or semi-complete (mechanical) destruction of adipose tissue and its original structure to obtain a mix of cells called "vascular fraction" or, better SVF (stromal vascular fraction), a preparation widely used in clinical and laboratory research but still subject to significant regulatory problems in standard clinical practice. The SVF obtained from a cc of adipose tissue contains several mesenchymal stem cells about 500 times greater than in cc of non-concentrated bone marrow aspirate. However, as we have seen, there is a poor correlation between the number of MSCs and biological/ clinical action, although the reasons for this behavior are still very unclear.

Bone marrow aspirate, lipoaspirate, MFAT, SVF, and expanded MSCs

From what has been said above, it is clear that Lipogems is not a device to isolate mesenchymal stem cells as many mistakenly believe mechanically. MFAT has nothing to do with SVF, which results from the enzymatic or mechanical breakdown of lipoaspirate with the destruction of the original tissue structure to obtain the possibility of isolating and possibly cultivating MSCs.

It is essential to understand the differences in the biological and clinical action of the different regenera-tive preparations: because a more significant number of MSCs not always translates into a more marked biological action, the same is valid for the secretome or exosomes obtained in vitro, and the in vivo measurement in experiment on animals [3] (fig. 2).

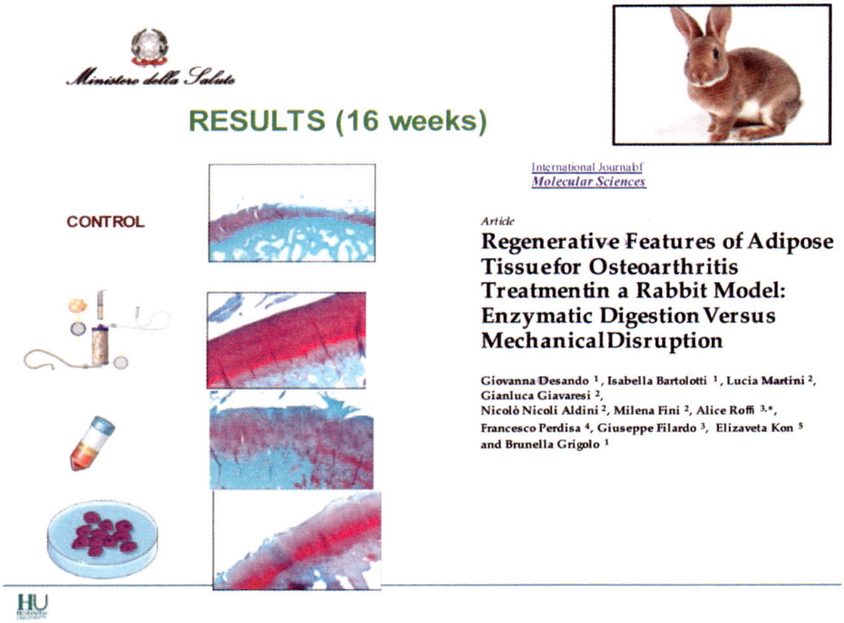

Figure 2 Experimental model on rabbit osteoarthritis where it is clear that there is absolutely no correlation between the number of MSCs and regenerative capacity since experimentally the quantitative differences in cartilaginous regeneration between MFAT, SVF and MSC cultivated are negligible, indeed, observing the histology it is noted that the neo-cartilage derived from MFAT is structurally more "normal" respecting all the natural maturation phases

The Lipogems device and why MFAT (lipogems) is structurally identical to lipoaspirate but with more effi-cient biological properties to be, in fact, an implantable natural bioreactor

The Lipogems system (fig 1c) was initially designed and patented by myself to optimize the clinical re-sults of lipofilling: the adipose tissue is sucked in by small disposable cannulas (14G) with multiple oval holes of 2x1mm (smaller holes slow down the procedure a lot and damage the sucked fat more). The aspi-rated adipose tissue, with a cluster size of about 3 mm, is inserted into a completely closed device that washes the fat from blood, oily and inflammatory residues. In the meantime, the size of the adipose clus-ter is gradually reduced to about 0.3 mm, through sharp filters and by only mechanical forces. For ensur-ing the correct processing [4], it is fundamental the absence of air so that the volumetric reduction is per-formed by exploiting the protection of the physiological pressure that avoids the destruction of adipo-cytes by burst while maintaining the structural integrity of the adipose tissue. The balls inside do not have the function of fragmenting the adipose tissue, but only to allow a good cleaning against the gravity of the oily emulsion/blood and to disperse the tissue so that it can be quickly passed through the second sharp filter. It is important to shake for no less than 20 seconds and 60 seconds in total, constantly checking the absence of air inside the device.

The product Lipogems (fig. 1 b) is the fragment of tissue *washed from oily impurities and dead cells and perfectly intact from the structural point of view* of about 300 microns (0.3mm) in diameter and repre-sents a fully functional *natural implantable bioreactor* that incorporates the main elements for a perfect natural regenerative response: the scaffold (the perfectly integrated structure also from the microvascular point of view of adipose tissue), cells (especially pericytes / MSC) and growth factors (secreted cytokines ini-

tially stimulated by mechanical trauma and later by the environment in which lipograms is implanted).
The local injection of such a tissue is a living graft, which easily integrates into the receiving tissue (the small size, less than 150/250 microns on each side, and the respect of the structure make it the ideal graft facilitating a rapid active and passive revascularization) and can work for a long time substantially im-proving the natural local healing potential.
In this regard, it is very interesting to note that in each of us, the recovery following a trauma or a disease is very different depending on the vascular micro density of the tissues [5], which varies inversely propor-tional to age and general conditions (for example in diabetic subjects a decrease in the vascular micro density, as well as in the tissue of the elderly compared to the child).
The reduction of the lipoaspirate from 3 mm to 0.3 mm in diameter causes a huge increase in grafted pieces. About 1,000 perfectly intact pieces are formed and covered on the surface by capillaries from each original fragment. The surface is even more increased (up to about 6,000 times), thus exposing a very large amount of capillaries and consequently of pericytes ready to function in a physiological way (fig. 1c). In addition, it has been shown that MFAT actively produces microcapillaries in vitro similar to the aor-ta ring and induces neovasculogenesis in the recipient tissue [6].
It is understandable how one of the primary mechanisms by which MFAT increases the healing capacity of tissues is to stably increase their vascular density, resulting in real tissue rejuvenation, as it is evident in particular by examining the histology of the treated tissues in gynecological and aesthetic applications even years after application (fig. 3 a, b)
The transplantation of microfracture adipose tissue according to the lipogems technique, which we will abbreviate as MFAT, has been used safely and effectively in tens of thousands of patients, in human and veterinary medicine, and in many different clinical applications for over 8 years [7].

The regulatory framework

The Lipogems device received FDA authorization in 2014 as a class II medical device for the processing of autologous adipose tissue. According to the FDA, Lipogems can be defined as a tissue:

- autologous;
- minimally manipulated;
- intended for homologous use (structural use);
- free of enzymes;
- not dependent on the metabolic activity of the cells for its primary function;
- used in the same surgical procedure
- not combined with anything other than saline.

In 2016 the FDA issued a second authorization to process adipose tissue for use in different surgical appli-cations, including arthroscopy: this means that MFAT is easily usable by the surgeon as an autologous transplant for musculoskeletal applications and within any joint. However, as the regulatory system of medical devices does not require it, *unlike drugs,*

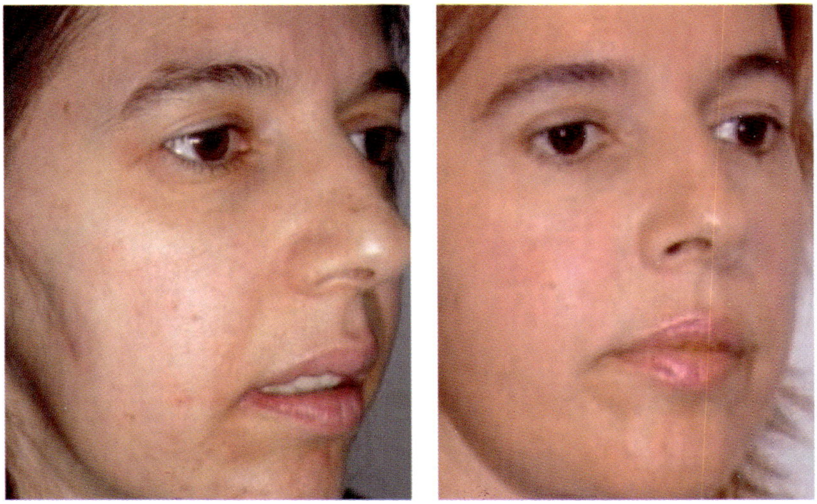

Figure 3 (A) Result at 8 years after two regenerative lipogems (at time 0 and after 5 years). Note the improvement of skin texture and vascularization in general that depend on the increase in vascular density of dermal tissues.

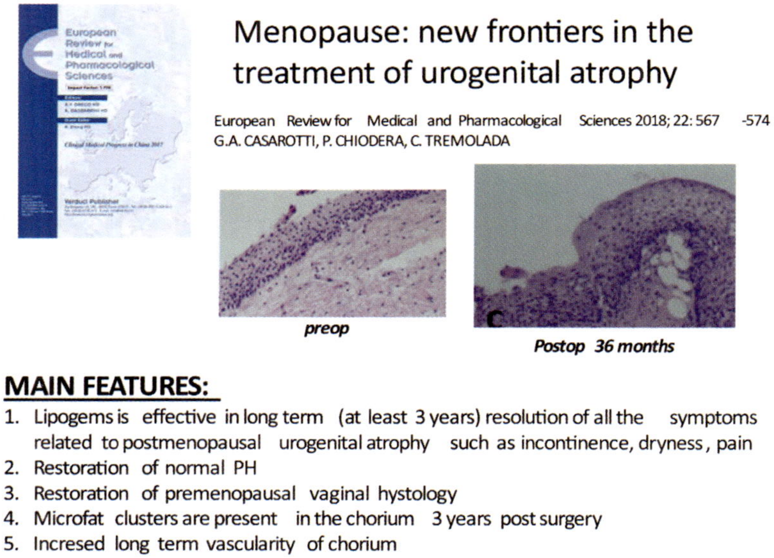

Figure 3 (B) Note the increase in vascular density in the chorion of the submucosa that causes the thickening of the vaginal mucosa and the presence of numerous glycogen granules in the cells that restore the correct Ph. Presence of cluster lipogems three years after the procedure. There is normally no adipose tissue in the mucous chorion.

there is no specific therapeutic indication of the device lipogems, for example for osteoarthritis; in addition, MFAT is considered by FDA, and EMA an autologous transplant and not a biological drug and the therapeutic indications are regulated by the rules of good medical-surgical practice that is by the indications derived from the results reported in clinical trials where the product lipogems / MFAT has been found safe and exceptionally effective [8].

Other devices for the processing of adipose tissue

Since Coleman presented his method for adipose tissue transplantation, there has been a proliferation of alternative methods and purported improvements. However, there is still no certainty on the best system to process fat due to the lack of methodologically flawless comparative trials and a sear-

Table 1

MOST USED TECHNIQUES FOR FAT GRAFTING

	Closed system	Cluster size	Quality of washing	Structural integrity	Ease of grafting
Lipogems	Yes	3 mm → 0,3 mm	++++	+++	++++ (the mini clusters are homogeneously dispersed in the fabric)
Coleman	No	3,5 mm	++	++	++
Megalon (SEFFI)	No	1.5 → 2 mm	+/-	++	+++
Tonnard (Nanofat/Tulip)	Yes/No	3 mm → ?? fat destruction	+/-	+/-	+/- (impossibility of tissue grafting)
Puregraft/ lipocell	Yes	4 mm/1.5 mm	++++	+++	++

ch of the articles published in the last year, that is, starting from 2020, has given over 3,000 results (table 1).

Clinical applications of Lipogems

In general surgery, Lipogems has been used as a valid approach for the treatment of fecal incontinence and fistulas, showing impressive morphological regeneration and long-term recovery of muscle and neuro-logical function even in irradiated soil [10].

In orthopedic surgery and better in the musculoskeletal field, most patients with degenerative and in-flammatory joint diseases can benefit from intra and peri-articular Lipogems with over 140 clinical articles in continuous updating [11].

After injecting a variable amount of Lipogems (2-12 ml depending on the joint), patients generally report-ed an evident and immediate improvement in symptoms but, above all, a long-term resolution of pain. In many cases, patients who were previous candidates for surgery, given the severity of the degeneration, no longer needed it due to the complete or substantial resolution of their symptoms. Radiographic and preoperative and postoperative MRI comparison showed in many cases a possible regeneration of articu-lar cartilage and an extension of joint space from 6 to 18 months after tre-atment; however, clinical im-provement is always more evident than radiographic improvement. In addition, lipogems or-thopedic use has also proven rewarding to promote repair in injured or degene-rated ligaments or tendons, in meniscal lesions, around surgical wounds, in and around osteotomy spaces.

These results have been confirmed in veterinary medicine where Lipogems is becoming an important re-genera-tive therapy in particular in dogs and horses but also exotic animals [12].

In reconstructive plastic surgery, Lipo-gems helps the healing of chronic ulce-ration of the legs and feet, especially in diabetic patients, with very encoura-ging results [13].

Cosmetic surgery is an ever-growing field of application, and Lipogems is used alo-ne or in association with traditional sur-gical techniques such as lifting, blepharo-plasty, breast augmentation, and others where the impression is that Lipogems improves and accelerates the time and quality of healing. Optimal results have been obtained in the periorbital area and orthognathic surgery. After surgery, pa-tients do not com-plain of pain, swelling, or bruising and are generally very sati-sfied with a continuous improvement of the skin texture and elasticity, parti-cularly evident from 9 to 18 postopera-tive months tracing quite faithfully what happens in other surgical fields where a powerful early anti-inflammatory effect is observed (hours/days) followed by a late and prolonged regenerative effect (months/years) [14].

Conclusion

Adipose tissue is the ideal source for extraction of mesenchymal stem cells, and above all for the clinical use becau-se it is easily accessible and collected through a minimally invasive surgical procedure, it can be found in sufficient quantities in most people and it guaran-tees an adequate amount of progenitor cells with good viability and a minimal-ly differentiating potential age-related. Lipogems technology naturally optimi-zes the healing and regenerative pro-perties of adipose tissue by reducing the size of adipose tissue clusters while maintaining their structural and functional integrity without using enzymes, additives, or centrifugations, but based on the use of mechanical forces and on the protection offered by the physiological that fills an entirely closed system in the absence of air.

Numerous randomized clinical trials are currently underway in different application fields to develop therapeutic strategies and innovative clinical protocols using different products derived from adipose tis-sue. We are convinced that a critical comparison between the different products is essential to identify which is the ideal preparation and the most homogeneous characteristics so that we can strategically concentrate clinical research efforts in this up-and-coming field.

References

1. https://scholar.google.com/scholar?hl=en&as_sdt=0,5&qsp=2&q=comparison+of+bone+marrow+%22adipose+tissue%22&qst=br.
2. https://scholar.google.com/scholaras_ylo=2020&q=msc+and+regeneration+mechanism&hl=en&as_sdt=0,5).
3. https://scholar.google.com/scholar?q=enzymatic+mechanical+adipose+tissue+processing+lipogems&hl=en&as_sdt=0%2C5&as_ylo=2015&as_yhi=
4. https://www.lipogems.com/lipogems-tutorial
5. https://scholar.google.com/scholar?hl=en&as_sdt=0%2C5&q=healing+capacity+vascular+density&btnG=
6. https://scholar.google.ch/scholar?hl=it&as_sdt=0%2C5&as_vis=1&q=lipogems+vasculogenesis&btnG=
7. https://scholar.google.ch/scholar?hl=it&as_sdt=0%2C5&as_vis=1&q=lipogems+mfat&btnG=
8. (https://scholar.google.com/scholar?hl=en&as_sdt=0%2C5&q=fda+lipogems&btnG=)
9. https://scholar.google.com/scholar?as_ylo=2020&q=processing+techniques+in+autologous+fat+grafting&hl=en&as_sdt=0,5
10. https://scholar.google.com/scholar?hl=en&as_sdt=0%2C5&as_ylo=2015&q=lipogems+and+mfat+in+colorectal+fistula+&btnG=
11. https://scholar.google.com/scholar?q=lipogems+and+mfat+in+orthopedics&hl=en&as_sdt=0%2C5&as_ylo=2015&as_yhi=
12. https://scholar.google.com/scholar?q=lipogems+and+mfat+in+veterinary+medicine&hl=en&as_sdt=0%2C5&as_ylo=2012&as_yhi=
13. https://scholar.google.com/scholar?hl=en&as_sdt=0%2C5&as_ylo=2012&q=lipogems+and+mfat+in+ulcers+and+diabetic+foot&btnG=
14. https://scholar.google.com/scholar?hl=en&as_sdt=0%2C5&as_ylo=2012&q=lipogems+and+mfat+in+aesthetic+and+orthognatic+surgery&btnG=